No Longer Radical

No Longer Radical

UNDERSTANDING MASTECTOMIES AND CHOOSING THE BREAST CANCER CARE THAT'S RIGHT FOR YOU

Rachel F. Brem, MD
Christy B. Teal, MD

SIMON ELEMENT

New York   London   Toronto   Sydney   New Delhi

SIMON ELEMENT

An Imprint of Simon & Schuster, Inc.
1230 Avenue of the Americas
New York, NY 10020

First Simon Element trade paperback edition May 2023

SIMON ELEMENT is a trademark of Simon & Schuster, Inc.

For information about special discounts for bulk purchases, please contact Simon & Schuster Special Sales at 1-866-506-1949 or business@simonandschuster.com.

The Simon & Schuster Speakers Bureau can bring authors to your live event. For more information or to book an event, contact the Simon & Schuster Speakers Bureau at 1-866-248-3049 or visit our website at www.simonspeakers.com.

Interior design by Silverglass

Manufactured in the United States of America

10 9 8 7 6 5 4 3 2 1

Library of Congress Control Number: 2022057975

ISBN 978-1-6680-0114-1
ISBN 978-1-6680-0113-4 (pbk)
ISBN 978-1-6680-0115-8 (ebook)

The names and identifying characteristics of all patients have been changed.

Mention of specific companies and organizations in this book does not imply endorsement by the authors or publishers, nor does it imply that such companies and organizations have endorsed the authors or publisher.

For my magnificent family, who fill my life with passion, inspiration, and love. And for everyone involved with the Brem Foundation: you make the world a better place.

—RFB

For Ashley, Nick, Ellie, and of course Dave.

—CBT

Contents

No Longer
Radical

CHAPTER 1

Are Mastectomies Right for You?

Everyone knows someone who has had breast cancer. And no wonder—one in eight American women are diagnosed in their lifetime. If that sounds terribly high, it is. In 2020, for the first time, breast cancer became the most common cancer in the world. As life spans have increased and a range of factors from diet to decreased childbearing to exposure to environmental contaminants have shifted, breast cancer has emerged as an all-too-common part of women's lives—and an all-too-common cause of their deaths. Fortunately, the odds of survival today are dramatically better than they were in the recent past. Major advances in genetic treatments, hormone therapy, and chemotherapy all give doctors, patients, and loved ones reason to be hopeful. Forty percent fewer women die of breast cancer now than two decades ago.

Although it has received less attention, another advance is at least as revolutionary—the shift in how we think about and perform mastectomies. They are safer and more effective than ever before, and reconstructive surgical techniques have advanced so rapidly that those who opt for breast reconstruction often marvel at how natural their new breasts look and feel.

What's more, women at high risk for cancer no longer have to endure the soul-crushing anxiety of hoping breast cancer doesn't happen—instead, they can intervene with preventive mastectomies.

If they have had cancer in one breast, they need not live in dread of getting cancer in the other one. If they're BRCA positive or have multiple first-degree family members with a history of breast cancer, they can preemptively remove their breasts. Instead of wishing, they can take action. Instead of hoping desperately to stay ahead of a disease we still don't fully understand, they can kick it out and bar the door.

Preventive mastectomies have become so popular that in recent years, three times as many women under age forty-five who are at increased risk of breast cancer have chosen to remove their healthy breasts. And as with so much in medicine, an ounce of prevention is worth a whole lot of cure. Advances in surgery now make it possible to have breast reconstruction during the same operation as mastectomies, so women can leave the operating room with new breasts of whatever size and shape they prefer and, if the surgery was prophylactic, with little to no risk of getting cancer. The relief women experience is often profound.

Studies show that when women have all their options presented clearly by a sympathetic doctor, they give mastectomies serious consideration, whether for treating breast cancer or preventing it. Yet the current trend in the medical community is to recommend that women attempt to save their natural breasts at all costs. Again and again our patients tell us how they were discouraged by their doctors from choosing mastectomies. The opposition was so strong that they felt they were not able to assess whether mastectomies were right for them or not.

Women diagnosed with breast cancer at a young age are increasingly opting for contralateral prophylactic mastectomies—i.e., removing the other, healthy breast—if their doctor leaves the option open. Doctors have a huge effect on their patients' choices and outcomes: women who discuss the option of mastectomies with a female surgeon are three times more likely to choose it than those who discuss it with a male surgeon.

In the past fifty years, our understanding and treatment of breast cancer has radically changed. We now know about close to eighty mutations associated with an increased risk for breast cancer, in addition to the well-known BRCA1 and BRCA2 mutations. More will undoubtedly be discovered. But knowing how we got to this point is also really important to understanding how much progress we've made.

In the 1970s, the best medical scientists considered breast cancer to be a viral infection. Suspecting that some cancers had a genetic component, Dr. Mary-Claire King relentlessly pursued her hunch for the next twenty-four years. Dr. King's identification of the BRCA1 and BRCA2 mutations in the early 1990s was a revolutionary breakthrough in understanding genetic risks for breast cancer: "There is no reason now that any woman with a mutation in BRCA1 or BRCA2 should ever die from breast or ovarian cancer," she said.[1] It's her view that identifying a woman as a carrier of a genetic mutation only after she develops cancer is "a failure of cancer prevention."[2]

More exciting innovations are constantly becoming available. We continue to improve methods for identifying those who are at an increased risk for breast cancer, as well as options to prevent breast cancer altogether. Mastectomies today are safe and highly effective in essentially eliminating the risk of getting breast cancer. That's an enormous relief to many women who are at a markedly increased risk of breast cancer. Of course, preventive mastectomies are not the right choice for every woman. Most women diagnosed with breast cancer can safely keep their breasts with minimal risk of recurrences or new cancers. But if you're at increased risk for developing breast cancer, or if mastectomy is right for you when breast cancer is diagnosed, or even if you're diagnosed with breast cancer that can be treated by a lumpectomy, we wrote this book to help educate you about your choices, so you can consider your options in an informed way and begin to open the conversation with your physician, family, and loved ones.

No matter where they live, or who their doctor is, women deserve to know that they may have access to a procedure that has brought relief, freedom, and even joy to both of us personally. As female doctors who have had mastectomies ourselves, we want to share with you the same critical information we give our patients every day. For decades, we've sat down with women to talk them through the facts, figures, and data they need to make the best decision for themselves. Too often, we're the first to tell them this option is even available.

We want to emphasize that the decision is a very personal one. The purpose of this book is to arm women with the information they need to make the right decision for themselves, a balanced decision based on all the latest medical and scientific updates. Not everyone at increased risk for breast cancer should undergo preventive mastectomies. However, *nobody* should be pushed or frightened into thinking that they should save their breasts at all costs. As is the case with nearly all decisions, there are pros and cons to both. After learning all the facts, the majority of our patients do not elect to do preventive mastectomies, but about 40 percent of them do, and they're very happy with the results.

Both of us—Rachel Brem, a breast radiologist, and Christy Teal, a breast surgeon—have been working in the trenches against breast cancer our entire careers. We've suffered devastating personal losses to breast cancer. And we're intimate with the uncertainties our readers face. We too struggled to decide: How high is our risk of breast cancer? Were we willing to live in suspense, anxious about every scan or test result? Would we actually go so far as to remove our breasts to eliminate cancer from our lives?

We each made different choices, as did the patients in the stories we'll share. Because we've both been grateful every day that we had mastectomies ourselves, we're in an ideal position—as individuals and as breast cancer doctors—to tell you exactly what to expect. We will walk you through the dozens of personal decisions you will be asked to make and help you figure out how to make them. It's essential to have information you can rely on when the choices are so critical and often made at a time of unfathomable stress. The decision will affect the rest of your life.

Preventive mastectomies can be one of the most positive, empowering ways for a woman to take control of her life by boldly and actively reducing her odds of getting breast cancer. And mastectomy to treat breast cancer can absolutely be the right decision for some women, even when conservative treatment where the breast could be saved is a safe medical option.

There is no right or wrong answer. Every person's decision is deeply personal and should be made on a case-by-case basis.

We're simply here to provide the insight and support that so many women want from their physicians but often do not receive. If you're considering having mastectomies because you have a genetic mutation, a strong family history of breast cancer, a diagnosis of breast cancer at a young age, postmenopausal breast cancer, or some combination of these, we hope to help you through the process of deciding what is best for you.

Rachel's Story

I always knew I wanted to be a doctor—a pediatrician, I thought. When I would go to my childhood doctor, I wanted to be that kind of person, someone who dedicated their life to helping others.

My plans changed after my mother's breast cancer diagnosis. My parents were immigrants—my mother was Israeli, my father initially from Poland. He was raised in a Siberian labor camp, forced there by the Russians. They met in Israel and instantly fell in love. Their love was extraordinary, and their devotion to each other and their family was unwavering. My mother was a vibrant whirlwind, and with her bright red hair and brilliant green eyes, her presence always filled our home with vitality. It was a shock to all of us when she was diagnosed with breast cancer at age thirty-three. I was twelve years old; my brothers were five and thirteen. She was told that she had six months to live. It was then that I decided I would dedicate my life to doing all I could so that other twelve-year-old girls and their families would not have to endure what we did.

My mother far outlived her doctors' predictions. But after her diagnosis, she was never quite the same. We lived on borrowed time with her, filled with gratitude but also worry about how much time she had left. After more than a decade in remission, she was diagnosed with ovarian cancer. I was in medical school at the time, and vowed to help her get the best treatment available.

She was one of the first patients to get what was then a new treatment—platinum-based therapy. Time has shown this approach to be very effective for BRCA-linked ovarian and breast cancers. Over the years, she had so many recurrences and metastatic sites that were treated with additional platinum-based therapy that she liked to say she had more platinum in her body than a jewelry store. She did everything she could to live, enduring round after round of chemo and other grueling interventions but never losing hope or the will to survive. Ultimately, she had ovarian cancer metastasize to her lung and underwent the excision of half her left lung. Miraculously, after additional chemotherapy, she never had cancer again. She was truly a miracle.

In the end, she died cancer-free at seventy-seven years old—forty-four years later than doctors predicted, although the numerous rounds of chemotherapy ravaged her body and undoubtedly contributed to her death.

That very first year, while my twelve-year-old mind was still staggering from the news, I announced to my parents that when I grew up, I was going to go to medical school to help find a cure for breast cancer. As touching as they must've found that sentiment, a "girl doctor" was a strange concept to them. They wanted their beloved daughter to *marry* a doctor, not to be one! They wanted me to have in my life what made them happy in theirs: a wonderful marriage, beautiful children, and friends who filled their home. But in the end, they loved that I was a doctor. They saw me dedicate my life to impacting others who had the disease that touched our family so deeply. They also saw that even as a doctor, I had those wonderful things in my life that they so cherished: a warm home, family, and friends.

As it turned out, I married a doctor, too. I met Henry Brem in synagogue while I was home from my first year of college. He was six years older than I, and a second-year Harvard Medical student. We grew up in the same little town in New Jersey: Fair Lawn, a haven for Jewish immigrants from Eastern Europe. Henry's sister, Shari, was my best friend from the age of seven. His parents were extraordinarily loving and committed. They were Holocaust survivors who had met in a displaced persons camp in Germany after being liberated from Nazi concentration camps by American troops. We all knew hardship. Breast cancer was always a big part of that narrative for our family. Early on in our courtship, I felt compelled to warn Henry that I, too, would likely get breast cancer. Although no gene had yet been identified, I was certain that breast cancer was my fate.

"I don't think that's what will happen," he said. "However, no matter what comes our way, we will handle it together!"

When I was nineteen, Henry and I married. Together we went through medical school, though at different times. He graduated from Harvard Medical School, and six years later, I graduated from the Columbia University College of Physicians and Surgeons. Our one-year-old daughter, Andrea, watched me walk across the stage to receive my diploma. It was the 1980s, and the first studies definitively demonstrating a mortality reduction from screening mammography were underway. I wanted to be part of that. I wanted to do all I could to minimize breast cancer deaths. I had my mother—that was not a given. I wanted other children to have theirs, too. I trained in radiology at Johns Hopkins. Alisa and Sarah, our twins, were born when I was a second-year radiology resident. Life was full and wonderful.

When I was thirty-seven, my maternal aunt was diagnosed with breast cancer, and I decided to be tested for the BRCA genetic mutation, which had recently been discovered. Very few women had been tested at that time, since the mutations had just been identified. I felt fortunate that I had the opportunity.

"If I have the mutation, I'll undergo preventive mastectomies," I told Henry. "If I don't, let's have another child."

The test confirmed it: I had the mutation—exactly as I had strongly suspected. But I could change my family's narrative. I could be there for my family and my patients. I could live to fulfill my dream of doing the research to introduce new and impactful approaches to decreasing the death rate from breast cancer.

Although preventive mastectomies were in their infancy, I thoroughly investigated the options. Henry and I traveled across the country meeting with breast and plastic surgical experts. When I decided where to have my surgery, I scheduled it for July 1996.

One evening, two weeks before my scheduled surgery, after a busy clinical day, I was trying a new ultrasound machine on myself to test image quality. Not only did I learn about this new machine—I also found my own breast cancer.

My intuition had been right all along.

Breast cancer has a timetable of its own. Although I had done everything possible to avoid getting breast cancer, I had just missed the window that would have made that possible.

I underwent bilateral mastectomies as scheduled, only they were no longer preventive; the surgery was to treat the breast cancer in one breast and undergo preventive mastectomy in the other. I also had my ovaries removed at that time. I had missed the chance to have preventive mastectomies, but was determined not to do the same with the ovarian cancer that ran in my family. My plan of having hormone replacement due to the surgical menopause from removing my ovaries was no longer possible, as women with breast cancer cannot take replacement hormones. However, I've been spared the difficulties of ovarian cancer. There is some comfort in the fact that there is now preliminary data to suggest that removal of the fallopian tubes (the tubes that connect the ovaries and the uterus) while leaving the ovaries in place may be enough to largely prevent ovarian cancer in women. It's not yet definitive, although the preliminary data is promising. Keeping your ovaries, not undergoing premature menopause, and even having additional children in the future may soon be shown to be possible for women with a genetic mutation that increases the risk of breast and ovarian cancers, even after having their fallopian tubes removed and thereby markedly decreasing the risk of ovarian cancer.

You don't need to have breast cancer to be a compassionate breast cancer physician. However, my experience, both growing up in a family touched in every way by breast and ovarian cancers, as well as being a breast cancer physician who went through the "breast cancer journey" myself, has given me a perspective that has positively impacted my practice and the care I provide my patients. I truly do use the yardstick of what would I want personally to advise and treat my patients, fully understanding that every patient has different needs and risks. Once again, there's a silver lining to my breast cancer cloud. Having had breast cancer has undoubtedly made me a better, more compassionate physician.

In the more than two decades since my surgery, I've profoundly benefited from the care I received and the choices I made. I've been privileged to share my life with Henry. We've raised three extraordinary daughters. We revel in our three incredible sons-in-law, and cherish, love, and laugh with our ten magnificent grandchildren. I am forever grateful for Henry's unwavering support and for the optimal care I received from my care team and my family.

Being a breast cancer doctor and having had breast cancer has shaped my choices and has motivated me to improve outcomes for women with breast cancer. Since early in my career, I've been dedicated to caring for women with breast cancer using the most advanced medical therapies and with the utmost compassion. My personal experiences have motivated me to focus on research to advance the field and develop better ways of diagnosing early, curable breast cancer.

This burning desire has resulted in my being part of the teams that have brought four new technologies to mainstream breast cancer care. I've published over 140 manuscripts in medical journals. I was the principal investigator for one of the first clinically available computer-aided detection devices for mammography.

This device increased the detection of early breast cancer by over 25 percent.

I was also part of the team that developed a molecular breast imaging technology that allows us to diagnose breast cancer based not only on how it looks but also how it functions. I worked with the team that developed the first FDA-cleared artificial intelligence for mammography that increases cancer detection, I was the principal investigator of the first multi-institutional study of automated whole-breast ultrasound to diagnose more early but aggressive cancers in women with dense breast tissue, and most recently I've been part of the team that discovered a game-changing FDA-cleared ultrasound technology: ultrasound tomography. Ultrasound tomography can detect additional early breast cancers in women with dense breasts, while decreasing the number of breast biopsies that are performed. This is also the first method of determining a woman's breast density without using ionizing radiation.

I've had the privilege of mentoring many medical students, residents, and fellows who have gone on to illustrious careers in which they have helped thousands of women, including those in underserved communities. My drive to improve outcomes from breast cancer is unrelenting. My hope is that we won't need these technologies in the future—when breast cancer is fully preventable.

Nearly twenty years ago, my patients and I noticed an enormous need for educating women from all socioeconomic backgrounds about the importance of early detection and risk-based personalized screening. In response to this need, we started the Brem Foundation to Defeat Breast Cancer. The Brem Foundation is dedicated to maximizing every woman's chance of finding an early, curable breast cancer through education, access, and advocacy. We've created an unprecedented curriculum for early detection that touches upon lesser-known but critical aspects of risk. The Brem Foundation uses in-person and digital forums for reaching women, and has created revolutionary programs to open access to care to underserved women. The foundation also educates physicians specializing in breast imaging. But we didn't stop there.

The Brem Foundation recognized that public policy is critical to moving the needle toward all women getting the care they need and deserve. That was why we wrote and helped to unanimously pass legislation in Washington, DC, that requires that women be informed about their breast density and that insurance cover essential screenings beyond mammograms for women with dense breast tissue and other risk factors. We're collaborating with national legislators to enact a national breast density notification law. We partnered with the ride-share company Lyft to offer underserved women cost-free rides to their mammograms, since free screening mammograms are ineffective if women cannot get to this lifesaving examination. We've developed award-winning educational videos that partner information and education with a lighthearted and fun (yes, fun) approach to educating women about breast cancer. You can see them yourself at bremfoundation .org. And we've only just begun. Perhaps best of all, my extraordinary daughter Andrea Wolf was the CEO of the Brem Foundation from 2015 to 2022 and was instrumental in bringing it to the level it has reached today. Andrea was a lawyer in DC before taking on this role. Her own decision to have prophylactic mastectomies at age thirty drew her to this work. Now she fights for a time when her four daughters will have better options to deal with their risks. Together, we're a mother-daughter team working tirelessly toward a world where far fewer women suffer from this sinister disease. Working with Andrea has been another breast cancer gift for me.

Breast cancer has been a difficult part of my life since I was twelve years old. But it has also been the source of my passion to improve the plight of breast cancer survivors—daughters, mothers, and wives. I got the BRCA gene and its resultant burdens from my mother, but she also instilled in me the passion to improve the plight of women with breast cancer. Breast cancer can indeed have a positive impact on one's life.

Only those who have experienced breast cancer can fully understand not only the medical impact but also the psychological and social impacts of being a breast cancer survivor. Similarly, only those who have a markedly increased risk of breast cancer understand the difficult decisions that must be made when knowledge of that risk comes to light: *How can I remove my healthy breasts to prevent a disease I don't have? If I have breast cancer and undergo conservative therapy, will I constantly be reminded that I was a cancer patient by the ever-present asymmetry of my breasts? How will this influence my decision to go to change in the gym locker room when my "cancer experience" is there for all to see? If I choose to keep my breasts, how do I live with the ever-present risk of a recurrence or a second cancer?*

Today, medicine has come so far with minimally invasive diagnoses and treatments that are extraordinary advances. However, as patients, we need to consider the consequences of less versus more aggressive approaches beyond initial treatment. It's the patient and her family who must live with the consequences of these monumental decisions.

With this book, Christy and I hope to inform and support an even wider group of women and their families with the information they need to make the best decisions for themselves.

Christy's Story

My first personal experience with breast cancer was in 1997 when my mother, age sixty, and my best friend Laurie, thirty-four, were diagnosed with breast cancer within a month of each other. Neither one had genetic mutations associated with breast cancer.

I was a new active-duty surgeon with the US Air Force at the time they developed breast cancers. When Laurie tested negative for a BRCA mutation, the results made me uneasy. I knew how far we had to go before we could say definitively that there was no genetic proclivity for breast cancer in anyone. Today, the National Institutes of

Health tracks more than twenty thousand variants of the BRCA1 and BRCA2 mutations,[3] but new mutations are being discovered every year. I believe without a doubt that Laurie's cancer was caused by a mutation that we simply haven't identified yet. Her father had died of breast cancer at forty-four—exactly ten years older than Laurie was when she was diagnosed. We have so much more to learn about our DNA and its endless mutations, so it's important to take a family history of cancer very seriously, despite a negative test. Sometimes it's the only warning sign.

While I felt certain that Laurie's cancer was caused by a genetic mutation that must not yet have been identified, I also supported her in her relief that her results were negative. She didn't want to have to think about the option of bilateral mastectomies back then. She was in a complicated relationship when she was diagnosed, but by the time her treatments were completed, the relationship had ended. Mastectomies were the last thing on her mind, and back in the 1990s, it was all so new. Even if she had tested positive, I'm not sure if mastectomies would have been the direction she would have gone at that time.

By comparison, my mother had an "easy" cancer. She had breast conservation surgery with a lumpectomy, sentinel lymph node biopsy, and radiation, then tamoxifen for five years. Since she was postmenopausal when she was diagnosed, I put the idea of my own risk of breast cancer out of my mind for years as I got on with my life: marrying, dedicating myself to my career as a surgeon, and raising three wonderful children.

The specter of cancer slipped into the background, until my mother came to town for the annual Race for the Cure in 2010. We celebrated her thirteen years of being cancer-free. As we walked, we both expressed how grateful we were that she had gotten off easily.

A few days after she'd returned home, she told me about a lump under her right arm that she had forgotten to mention when she was visiting. I was relieved, since her cancer had been in her left breast. I assumed it would be nothing and, indeed, a mammogram and ultrasound at the local hospital didn't show anything in her right breast. I wanted to be sure, and recommended that she have the lump biopsied. A few days later, she called me with the results—the lymph node showed metastatic cancer from the breast. She came to the George Washington University Hospital so Rachel could do additional scans.

When she looked at my mother's MRI, Rachel saw the cancer in her right breast and in many of her lymph nodes. We were devastated that cancer was back in the picture, this time in the other breast—and much more aggressive. To me, it behaved like a cancer caused by a genetic mutation.

Based on the MRI, it appeared that my mother would need a mastectomy, and she decided to have both breasts removed. She didn't feel it was worth trying to match her right breast to the left, which was already abnormal-looking from her prior cancer treatment. My colleague Dr. Anita McSwain agreed to do my mother's bilateral mastectomies and right lymph node dissection. She took amazing care of her, and of my father. She was also honest with me that there were going to be many lymph nodes involved, based on what she felt at the time of surgery. My mother recovered well, but the whole process was much harder than it had been the first time. We knew that chemotherapy and chest wall radiation were going to be necessary.

Not long afterward, Rachel pulled me aside and asked, "When are you going to have your own mastectomies?" It was as if she had read my mind. I had always thought I'd wait until I had some sign of cancer, but thinking about how aggressive my mother's new cancer was, I was starting to reconsider, especially since her cancer could not be found on a mammogram or ultrasound. I had always known that if I were ever diagnosed with breast cancer, I would likely have bilateral mastectomies, especially after nipple-sparing mastectomies became an option. I knew that the data showed that for women diagnosed with breast cancer, having a mastectomy doesn't improve your chances of survival, but I also knew that with mastectomies, I wouldn't need to worry about additional imaging. More important, I knew that bilateral mastectomies would reduce my risk for ever developing breast cancer to 1 to 2 percent, odds that were attractive to me. In addition, my breasts were always small, but became even more so after breastfeeding my three children, so the cosmetic result of breast conservation if I ever developed breast cancer might not be ideal. With implants, I would end up with beautiful, shapely breasts, and nipple-sparing mastectomies resulted in amazing cosmetic results. If I were to be diagnosed with breast cancer, the choice seemed clear. Why not do it when I was in complete control and could prevent cancer altogether?

My mother's meetings with the genetic counselor revealed that one of her aunts had died from breast cancer in her early fifties. We only learned about this when she reached out to her cousin. Since there were very few other women in the family, I was even more worried that there may be a genetic predisposition, even though my mother's genetic test came back negative. Repeat testing in 2015 after her cancer recurred was still negative.

When I decided it was time to schedule my preventive mastectomies, I knew my choice would likely be controversial. But I knew that it was the right decision for me, and my husband, Dave, agreed. My mother was immediately supportive. After her diagnosis in 2010, she felt pretty sure she would ultimately die of breast cancer. She wanted me to do whatever it took to avoid that fate.

While many colleagues were understanding and supportive, others gave a response we still hear today: preventive mastectomies are only recommended for women with genetic mutations. Many told me that since my mother's test came back negative and my mammogram was normal, I didn't need to consider having mastectomies.

I was frustrated that so many physicians told me I didn't need to have the surgery that I knew was right for me. It made me wonder how many other women exploring the option were being told the exact same thing. I felt that I needed to share my story to let others know that it's not a wrong choice, just a personal one. I contacted Cindy Rich, a reporter from the *Washingtonian*, and invited her to follow me through the process, from making the decision to have mastectomies and the type of reconstruction I wanted. I wanted her to reach other women considering mastectomies and their families to let them know that while mastectomies may not be the right option for many women, they're a reasonable option for others.

Shortly prior to the publication of the *Washingtonian* article in July 2011,[4] I was invited to appear on *Good Morning America.* Robin Roberts interviewed me a week after my expander exchange surgery on a show entitled "Confronting a Family History of Breast Cancer, a Surgeon Makes a Radical Decision."[5] But I didn't believe that it was radical then, and I certainly don't believe it is now. To this day, I'm touched and proud of my efforts when women tell me they saw my interview or read the article and are thankful for the information and validation for the procedures they're considering. I often tell my patients who are having preventive mastectomies that they're beating cancer before ever getting it. With this book I hope we can reach even more women.

My mother's cancer recurred in 2014. When it progressed in 2016, we decided to take a vacation abroad. She had always wanted to show my daughters London and Paris. She and my father had taken the other grandchildren on special trips, usually in groups of two or three at a time when they were young teenagers. We all knew this was likely to be her last trip with her grandchildren, and I was thrilled that I was invited to join her and the girls. She was not as energetic as usual. At the time, I blamed it on chemotherapy, but we now know that it was from the cancer taking over her body. That she was able to go on every single tour and enjoy every meal was amazing, knowing what I know now. She was truly remarkable.

As we stood in line at the Eiffel Tower on our last day in Paris, the girls were complaining about having to wait so long. It had been a long day for all of us. I asked my mother what she wanted to do. She answered, "I don't think I will be back here again, so I would like to go to the top." We did, and it was worth it. I treasure the photos and incredible memories.

Once we got home, she declined rapidly. Additional tests were done, which showed the cancer had spread. When she could not keep down food, she was admitted to the hospital. Not long afterward, my older brother called to say that she was not doing well. We moved her to inpatient hospice, which was her wish. We all felt lucky that we could be with her in the end, with dignity and her usual grace. My younger brother and his family visited her just after she was placed in hospice, when she could still communicate well. My older sister and brother were there already. By the time my family was able to see her, she could hear us but could barely speak. The kids and I hugged her and held her hands. She gave me my fiftieth birthday present, a necklace she had made with her mother's engagement diamond, knowing that she would not be here for my birthday in November. I wear it almost every day, and treasure it. When I touch it, I feel her presence.

Even though she knew cancer would catch up with her eventually, my mother had hoped to reach eighty. "After eighty, it's all downhill anyway!" she said. She didn't quite make it, but lived to be seventy-nine, long enough to spend many precious years with her husband, children, and beloved grandchildren. I often reflect that if her first cancer had been as aggressive as her second, she would never have met my children. It's such a gift that they had the chance to know her. The other gift is that as soon as she was in hospice, my siblings, their spouses, and their children were able to be there with her and my father when she was in her final moments. It was as peaceful as we could have hoped.

The decision to have preventive mastectomies—with or without cancer, with or without known genetic mutations—could not be more important to me, both personally and professionally. That's why I wanted to write this book with Rachel. My older brother once asked me if my mother would still be with us today if she had had bilateral mastectomies when she was first diagnosed. Of course, we don't know the answer to that, but she would definitely not have died from breast cancer. I had mastectomies, so I will never have to wonder if that will be my fate.

CHAPTER 2

High-Risk Screening

Because of the incredible strides in early detection of breast cancer and targeted and novel therapies, the death rate from breast cancer has declined by *almost half* in the past twenty years.[1] Most women (63 percent) are diagnosed before the cancer has metastasized, or spread to other parts of the body. The five-year survival rate for early breast cancer is greater than 95 percent.[2] We've seen major advances in diagnosis, treatment, and screening. Now the question is, how do I screen for breast cancer, understanding that *every* woman is at risk, and that breast cancer found early is curable? Screening for breast cancer has become far more personalized in recent years. It's no longer assumed that every woman should be screened with only a mammogram every year. So how can you make sure you're getting the care you need?

TWO PRIMARY CRITERIA

We now routinely adjust surveillance, or screening, for breast cancer based on two primary criteria: your breast density and your risk of getting breast cancer.

Breast density is determined by the amount of glandular tissue in a breast. It's a strong risk factor for developing breast cancer.

Currently, the only way to know if you have dense breast tissue is to see how much white tissue there is on your mammogram.

Women with dense breast tissue, like all women over age forty, must have an annual mammogram to detect early, curable breast cancer. The challenge is that on a mammogram, breast tissue is white and breast cancer is white. Therefore, the ability to detect breast cancer with a mammogram is significantly diminished in women with dense breasts. What is even more daunting is that the risk for developing breast cancer is up to four times higher in women with dense breasts.[3]

Overall, mammography detects 85 percent of breast cancers, but in women with dense breasts, that decreases to between 45 and 65 percent.[4] Although this is disappointing, it's critical to remember that mammography still finds most cancers in women with dense breasts, and it remains an important component of screening for breast cancer.

If you have dense breasts, there are additional ways to look for cancers that are hidden in mammograms. MRI can certainly find these cancers. So can screening breast ultrasound, the same ultrasound that's used to image babies in utero, which doesn't use ionizing radiation. In fact, on an ultrasound, dense tissue is white and breast cancer is dark, so the ability of ultrasound to detect breast cancer in women with dense breasts is actually better. That being said, there are certainly still cancers that can be seen only through mammography, even in women with dense breast tissue.

If the report given to you by the radiologist indicates that you have dense breasts, you should insist on an annual screening breast ultrasound. Numerous studies, including some that we had the privilege of leading, have shown that in women with dense breasts, ultrasound can find up to 25 percent more cancers.[5] That alone is a great stride forward. Furthermore, the types of cancer that ultrasound finds in women with dense breasts are clinically critical cancers—small, early, invasive breast cancer. These are the cancers we *must find* to save lives, because they have the propensity to metastasize and become killers.

It's critical that women with dense breast tissue have annual screening ultrasounds in addition to annual screening mammograms to optimize their ability to detect early, curable breast cancers.

THE POLITICS OF BREAST DENSITY

The issue of breast density isn't only medical but political. Women deserve the right to know about the importance of breast density. In 2018, twenty-nine states had laws that required an indication of a woman's breast density be part of the letter that's sent to her with her mammography results. In 2022, thirty-seven states and the District of Columbia had breast density notification laws, and a federal bill was introduced in Congress that year.

Where we work with and care for women in the District of Columbia, the death rate from breast cancer is the highest in the country. In response to this, Andrea Wolf, CEO of the Brem Foundation to Defeat Breast Cancer, helped write and pass the Breast Density Screening and Notification Amendment Act of 2018 (DC Law 22-261), which requires doctors to inform women of their breast density and insurance companies to cover not only ultrasound but also MRI and any future technologies to screen for cancer in women with dense breasts. Not only did the bill unanimously pass but DC went further and, with the support of the Brem Foundation, included the requirement that insurance companies provide mandatory coverage of the cost of the lifesaving additional annual ultrasound and other screening imaging studies for women with dense breast tissue.

Andrea's vision and commitment to improving outcomes for women has resulted in her initiating a movement to change the wording of adjunct screening for women with dense breasts from "additional" to "essential screening," since that's what it is, and now the terminology that's increasingly being used reflects this.

This was not enough for Andrea and the team at the Brem Foundation. For many underserved women, free mammography was not enough. There was an enormous barrier to obtaining lifesaving mammography: although one of the benefits of the Affordable Care Act was no-cost mammograms, underserved women often didn't have the means to get to appointments. The Brem Foundation partnered with the ride-share company Lyft to develop a program to break down the barrier for under-resourced women called Wheels for Women, providing no-cost-to-them rides to their free mammograms. This program has been a resounding success and is being utilized by many more women than expected. Women's lives are truly being saved by the breast density notification bill, the Wheels for Women program, and the change in language from "additional" to "essential" screening.

Anne K. is a successful writer who's committed to living the healthiest lifestyle she can. She was deeply impacted by the fact that her mother had breast cancer. Anne also has dense breast tissue. Following a normal mammogram that showed her dense breast tissue, she had an annual screening ultrasound that demonstrated a small, highly aggressive breast cancer. She was shocked but also deeply grateful for the additional testing. She decided to take this opportunity to help others benefit from annual screening ultrasound. So when the Brem Foundation asked her to join them to testify before the Council of the District of Columbia (DC's city council) to enact the bill the foundation had written and proposed, she enthusiastically participated. Anne took a life challenge and used it to improve, and indeed, save, the lives of many others.

Today, thirty-seven states and the District of Columbia have passed breast density notification legislation requiring that women be informed of their breast density. However, these laws are all different: some simply tell a woman she has dense breasts; some include information about other imaging modalities, such as ultrasound and MRI, that can find additional cancers that are hidden on mammography; and some require insurance coverage of the additional testing. Once again, breast cancer isn't only a medical condition but a political one, that hopefully will further empower women with the knowledge they need to advocate for and seek the care they deserve.

Whether you have perky or saggy breasts doesn't determine if you have dense breasts. Half of American women have fatty, non-dense breast tissue; the other half have dense breast tissue.[6] In this case, fat is good. The fattier your breasts are, the easier it is to interpret your mammograms. Today, only a mammogram can determine your breast density. Excitingly, the FDA recently approved a new method to determine breast density without radiation. Developed by Delphinus Medical Technologies, this technology is known as SoftVue ultrasound tomography.

MAMMOGRAMS

Not all mammograms are the same. The newest technology is 3D mammography, or tomosynthesis. While 2D mammography shows a picture of the breast, 3D mammography shows images of slices or layers through the breast. That provides a significant advantage. Sometimes overlapping breast tissue hides cancer behind it with 2D images—3D mammography helps with that problem.

Every woman will get better results with 3D mammograms, but for women with dense breasts, the advantages of 3D mammography are even better, with a slightly higher breast cancer detection rate and a lower rate of unclear findings that require women to return for additional mammographic evaluation (known as callbacks).

There are potential risks from mammography, including the radiation required for the examination. However, it's important to
realize that your exposure to radiation on a flight across the US is
greater than your exposure during a mammogram, and there's absolutely no evidence that mammography has ever resulted in a single
breast cancer. Nearly all physicists believe that there's a threshold
for the negative impact of radiation. That means that unless you're
exposed to radiation above a threshold that's far higher than dozens
of mammograms, the impact of the radiation is essentially zero and
harmless. Therefore, with all the discussions of the pros and cons of
mammography, the pros far outweigh any potential harm.

Screening Mammogram

- If you have no signs of breast cancer—no lump, no palpable
  findings, no new nipple discharge, no skin thickening, and no
  lesions—you can have a screening mammogram. Screening
  mammography is covered with no co-pay or deductible under
  the Affordable Care Act (ACA), so it's free to the patient. Even
  if it's early in the year and you haven't yet met your deductible,
  screening mammograms are free! This isn't the case with a
  diagnostic mammogram, which is performed for women with
  signs or symptoms of breast cancer. A diagnostic mammogram
  may well be covered by your insurance, but not without the
  deductible and co-pay of your individual insurance plan. Even
  if you've had a normal screening mammogram, if you develop
  a finding or a symptom between screening mammograms, you
  should have a diagnostic mammogram.
- With screening mammograms, whether 2D or 3D, you might
  get asked to return for additional imaging to get a clearer
  picture of what the radiologist found on your mammogram,
  what we refer to as a "callback." Ten to 15 percent of women
  undergoing screening mammography are called back for more

imaging. If you're called back, it doesn't mean you have breast cancer. Rather, it means the radiologist found something on your mammogram that needs additional evaluation. With 3D mammography, fewer women are called back. By law, you must receive the results of your screening mammogram within thirty days of your exam in writing and in "lay terms," meaning language that everyone should understand. It should also tell you what your next steps are, such as another mammogram in a year, or additional imaging if there was an unclear area on your screening mammogram.

- It's important to note that if you're called back, the additional imaging is likely to determine that there is no cancer. So don't fret if you get a call or a letter saying you need to return for more studies. Instead, think of it as an insurance policy to make sure you don't have breast cancer. Generally, a few additional images or an ultrasound will clear things up. And if the imaging does find cancer, that's the purpose of mammography—the opportunity to find early, curable breast cancer.

- After a suspicious finding, a biopsy may be needed to determine whether you have breast cancer. Today, all breast biopsies should be minimally invasively, performed with a needle, not a scalpel. The biopsy is similar in severity to going to the dentist. Local anesthesia is used to numb the area. There are no stitches, and many women return to their daily routine directly from the biopsy.

- As scary as it may seem, rest assured that the results of over 80 percent of breast biopsies are benign. (We will have more to say about breast biopsies later.)

Diagnostic Mammogram

- A diagnostic mammogram is recommended if you have any signs or symptoms of breast cancer, such as a new lump, new nipple discharge, a lesion on your nipple, or dimpling of the skin on your breast. A radiologist will review the images as they're taken, order any additional imaging, and, if needed, recommend a biopsy. You should get the results of your breast imaging on the same day. Of course, if you do need a biopsy, it will take up to a week, or sometimes more, to get the results.

- Often, a suspicious or unclear finding can be resolved by comparing the current mammogram to your prior mammograms, so it's a good idea to bring any prior mammograms with you to your appointment if you had the imaging performed at a different institution. If you go to the same place for your mammogram every year, they will have your prior images. If you had mammograms at other institutions, make sure to bring a disc with the images, not just the prior reports, since reports alone won't be adequate for comparison.

MRIs

MRI is often needed to screen women who have a personal history of breast cancer, who previously had radiation therapy for lymphoma, or who have a finding of atypia on a breast biopsy. Additionally, women with a history of breast cancer in multiple family members or a personal history of breast cancer, especially premenopausal breast cancer, should consider having screening MRIs. Women with a mutation that substantially increases their risk of breast cancer, such as BRCA1, BRCA2, or any of the other increasingly identified mutations associated with a marked increase in risk of breast cancer, need annual MRI screening. The American Cancer Society now recommends that women with a lifetime risk for breast cancer of 20 percent or greater should have a yearly breast MRI, which should be done with intravenous contrast, in addition to annual mammography, since it offers the best way to see the earliest cancer. In some women, annual screening mammography along with screening breast ultrasound is needed to detect early, curable breast cancer. How you or your doctor determines your risk is discussed in the section on risk assessment in chapter 3. Note that not all physicians recommend MRIs for all high-risk women and not all insurance companies cover the study, so check with your insurer. Some doctors may not think MRI is needed, even for high-risk women. If you're at substantially increased risk of breast cancer, you should advocate for yourself and insist on additional MRI imaging for the best chance to find early, curable breast cancer.

Understandably, patients often ask us whether they should have an MRI even if they don't have an increased risk of breast cancer, since it's the most sensitive test for detecting early cancer. There are a few reasons we don't recommend this.

All MRI examinations for breast cancer require an injection with a contrast agent (commonly gadolinium). The contrast is injected into your arm and then circulates in your blood, allowing the radiologist interpreting the images to see areas in the breast to which there is more blood flow. In addition, the uptake of the contrast in breast tissue is different depending on the tissue type, with cancer taking up more contrast soon after injection and normal tissue taking up less contrast and later. We use this difference to find the smallest cancers with the greatest accuracy. Unlike mammography and ultrasound, which evaluate how tissues look, contrast allows us to evaluate how tissues function and in more detail. This difference makes MRI more sensitive for the detection of cancer. With MRI and some other tests, like molecular breast imaging (MBI) and contrast-enhanced spectral mammography (CESM), we see not only how tissues look but how they act, similar to MRI.

There are some concerns with the repeated injection of

gadolinium-based contrast agents. Some women may simply not want to get an injection every year for a screening test, which is understandable. From a medical perspective, in 2017, the FDA issued a new warning when they learned that gadolinium—a heavy metal—accumulates in the brain and stays for months or even years.[7] They haven't found any evidence of harm from gadolinium or its accumulation in the brain, but we still would like to minimize the amount of heavy metals in the body.

An important note: When reviewing the results of breast MRI examinations, it's important to be aware that the test can result in a false positive. MRI can show benign masses such as fibroadenomas or other findings that may lead to a biopsy. The tissue taken at the time of the biopsy is examined by a pathologist to determine if it's cancer. Eighty percent of biopsies are not cancer (benign), but we have to examine the concerning areas seen on the study to find the smallest breast cancer. So although MRI is the most sensitive way to find breast cancer, it must be used judiciously.

OPTIMAL SCREENING

For Women

One thing is certain. If you're a woman age forty or over, you should get a screening mammogram every year, as long as you have no symptoms. If you do have symptoms or develop them between mammograms, insist on a diagnostic mammogram right away. You absolutely should not wait until your next annual mammogram.

In the medical community, everyone agrees that women should be screened. After that, things get dicey.

The guidelines of different organizations vary. The only thing that's certain about this advice is that these organizations can't agree.

The US Preventive Services Task Force recommends that women age fifty to seventy-four get a mammogram every other year. This reduces the odds of mortality by 81 percent. Since 19 percent more women die of their disease from not getting a mammogram every year starting at age forty, we strongly encourage and recommend that women begin screening at age forty and not at fifty, and get a mammogram every year.

The American Academy of Family Physicians urges women to start screening annually at age fifty and get a mammogram every other year.

The American Cancer Society prefers that women from age forty to forty-four have annual screenings but says they can wait until they're forty-five to start. Once they're fifty-five, they should have mammograms every year or every other year until their life expectancy is ten years or less.

Why doesn't the American Cancer Society recommend annual screening mammography for average-risk women age forty and above? Because of the potential "harms of mammography." The greatest harm described is the anxiety women feel over a false positive finding—that is, a mammogram that has a finding that ultimately is determined not to be cancer—that requires additional screening with a diagnostic mammogram, ultrasound, or MRI. Certainly, getting called back for additional imaging after a screening mammogram will cause a woman to be concerned, even anxious. However, studies have unequivocally demonstrated that the anxiety from a positive mammogram is real, but it's transient and has no long-term effect.[8]

As physicians who have cared for women with breast cancer for decades, we assure you that the anxiety a woman feels when she returns for additional testing is real, but it's far less anxiety than she will feel if she's told she has incurable metastatic breast cancer. We're all about empowering women. We strongly believe that women should have the opportunity to have the earliest, most curable breast cancers detected, and that means starting at age forty for women of average risk for breast cancer. It's astonishing to us as women and as physicians that some organizations are using anxiety as an excuse to discourage lifesaving screening mammography. We should make that decision ourselves.

When a woman is diagnosed with more advanced breast cancer and is cured due to the ever-improving therapies over the past decades, the journey she has to endure to achieve that cure—what we call her "intensity of care"—is far more involved and difficult than the journey of a woman diagnosed with an earlier breast cancer. Women deserve to advocate for themselves and get the best care with the best outcome and the lowest intensity of care. It's every woman's right. If there's one message to take away here, it's that you must insist on getting a mammogram *every year* beginning at age forty to optimize your opportunity to find early, curable breast cancer.

For Women at Increased Risk

The best recommendations for breast cancer screening take a woman's individual risk into consideration for women:

- **Age forty or over.** A mammogram every year.
- **Dense breasts.** A mammogram and ultrasound every year.
- **First-degree relative with breast cancer.** Start screening ten years earlier than the age at which that relative was diagnosed.
- **Genetic mutation (or greater than 20 percent lifetime risk of breast cancer).** MRI every year separated by six months from an annual mammogram. If you have a genetic mutation that's associated with a substantially increased risk of breast cancer, then you should begin annual MRI at age twenty-five and annual 3D mammography at age thirty.
- **Unusual findings (atypia) or prior history of breast cancer (15 to 19 percent increase).** Consider having an MRI every year between mammograms.

For women at intermediate lifetime risk of breast cancer—that is, those who have a 15 to 19 percent lifetime risk—your risk tolerance may impact your decision to have annual screening MRI. It's clear that in women with a personal history of breast cancer who have had lumpectomy or women who have had a biopsy that has demonstrated atypia (abnormal cells), annual MRI finds substantially more cancers. Moreover, a recent study from the Netherlands reported that in women with extremely dense breast tissue, annual screening MRI finds substantially more cancers than mammography and ultrasound. What does that mean for you? It depends on your risk tolerance. If your approach is to do all you can to find the earliest of cancers, annual screening MRI is extremely helpful. However, the more MRIs you have, the more likely you are to have a false positive, a finding that requires additional evaluation or even possibly a minimally invasive biopsy, and the greater your exposure to gadolinium-based contrast agents.

For Women of Color
The American College of Radiology considers women of color to be a high-risk group. All women, including women of color, should begin annual screening at age forty, but studies have recently demonstrated that women of color get 3D mammography at a much lower rate than other women, and their time from diagnosis to treatment is much longer.[9] Women of color have a 40 percent higher death rate from breast cancer compared to Caucasian women. This is due to a combination of factors, including limited access, lower participation in clinical trials that allow for more targeted genomic therapy, and biological differences, since women of color have triple-negative breast cancer (the most aggressive kind) more often.

As healthcare providers, we must first recognize this unacceptable statistic, then do all we can to work together to minimize and hopefully eliminate this disparity. We must be committed to ensuring that communities of color have access not only to screening and treatment for breast cancer but also to high-quality care. We cannot accept anything less.

For Women with Bilateral Prophylactic Mastectomies

If you've had bilateral prophylactic mastectomies, you've reduced your risk of breast cancer by 95 percent. The number of annual screenings you need is none.

You do need to continue to do self-examinations, and if you feel something questionable, seek a doctor's advice. If you've had reconstruction with silicone implants, continue to do an MRI without contrast, as contrast isn't needed to evaluate implants, every three to five years to assess the integrity of the implants. Otherwise, you don't have to worry about it.

For Men

We cannot end our discussion of screening for breast cancer without addressing the needs of men who have a genetic mutation with a markedly increased risk of breast cancer. As we know, not all genes that result in an increased risk of breast cancer are the same. Men with a BRCA2 mutation have the highest risk of breast cancer, about the same risk as a woman without the mutation.[10] It's recommended that men with a BRCA2 mutation have annual screening mammography. Since men rarely have dense breasts, that should be sufficient, unless a mammographic or clinical finding warrants additional evaluation with ultrasound.

The recommendations for men with other genetic mutations that increase the risk of breast cancer are less clear. Only 1 percent of breast cancer occurs in men. Therefore, all men, whether they have genetic mutations with increased breast cancer risk or not, should be vigilant. If they feel a breast mass, they should see a doctor.

Breast cancer screening is increasingly being called for by the transgender community. If transgender men have had bilateral mastectomies, screening isn't needed. If they haven't, annual screening is recommended. For transgender women, if they have been on hormonal therapy for more than five years, then annual screening mammography is recommended.

Overall, the good news is that the death rate from breast cancer has decreased by 40 percent over the past twenty years. Screening accounts for about half of this reduction.[11]

If there's one message to take away from this chapter, it's that you must insist on an annual mammogram beginning at age forty if you're at average risk of breast cancer. If you have dense breasts or have other reasons for increased risk, then you should have additional screening with ultrasound or MRI. We must do all we can to optimize the detection of early breast cancer so that after diagnosis, women can have the best outcome with the lowest intensity of care. Breast cancer screening protocols must be personalized and based on a woman's risk for breast cancer as well as her breast density and risk tolerance. Do that, and whatever your risk, you will be improving the odds in your favor.

Common Questions to Discuss with Your Care Team

Do I need to have screening breast ultrasound in addition to a mammogram every year?

Should I get a mammogram every year?

How are MRIs different from mammograms? Do they use radiation?

When should I start getting mammograms?

Is my mammogram covered by insurance?

What's the difference between a screening mammogram and a diagnostic mammogram?

Does my radiologist specialize in breast imaging?

Can I get a mammogram if I have breast implants?

Is there one test for breast cancer that's best?

I thought if my mammogram was normal, it meant I didn't have breast cancer. Is that true?

What are the different types of mammograms?

If I have a screening mammogram and am told I need to return for additional imaging, does that mean I have breast cancer?

Does it matter when during my menstrual cycle I get my mammogram?

I find mammograms quite painful. Is there anything I can do to minimize the discomfort?

Are mammograms dangerous?

Does getting a mammogram make a difference?

Am I too young for breast cancer?

Should I get a clinical breast examination from my doctor?

CHAPTER 3

Pathology, State-of-the-Art Treatment & Recovery

NOTE TO READERS: This chapter is meant as a reference guide for the different types of breast cancers and therapeutic regimens for women who have already been diagnosed with cancer. Women who had preventive mastectomies before they had cancer can skip this chapter.

Many of our cancer patients are surprised that they need treatment after surgery. Removing cancerous tumors or an entire breast is only one step in the treatment of breast cancer. We want to make sure that all the cancer is gone. The tumor may have been in one location, but it emerged in the environment of your body, where the cells can be in other places in the body. Though the cancerous cells were primarily focused in one place, and we remove as many of them as we can, there may be more cancerous cells in the surrounding tissue or circulating in your blood on a microscopic level.

We can't go in and remove each breast cancer cell, so we may follow surgery with chemotherapy and/or hormonal therapy with the goal of completely eliminating the cancer (chemotherapy is also sometimes given before surgery). Radiation may be part of the treatment as well. All of this likely sounds confusing. But cancer care is individualized; there's no one size fits all. However, you will have a team of people from many different specialties taking care of you and guiding you every step of the way. The key is to pick the team that's right for you. We're here to help with that as well.

Breast cancer is actually not one single disease. Rather, it's hundreds or even thousands of different types of disease, and there's no one treatment that's effective for everyone. Many different analyses and treatments are used to determine the best treatment for you and to treat your breast cancer, depending on what kind of breast cancer is being treated, the stage at diagnosis, and how well it responds to treatment. Your breast surgeon and medical oncologist will talk you through the steps. This chapter is meant to give you more insights into those discussions and help ensure that you come away with a clear understanding of your options. While it's very technical, it will be especially useful to refer to as you navigate your treatment options and what you can expect as a result.

Don't feel like you have to read about every different type of cancer and treatment. It can be overwhelming. Instead, we recommend that you focus on the parts of the chapter that relate to the diagnosis that concerns you; we've used a lot of subheadings and bullets to make the text easier for you to scan. Of course, all the information presented in this chapter is here to help you feel confident that you know how to get the best care for your unique situation.

PATHOLOGY

When you're diagnosed with breast cancer, it's helpful to look at a diagram of a breast so you can see where the cancer cells are developing.

Your breast is made up of lobules where milk is made and ducts that take the milk to the nipple in women who are nursing. More cancers develop in the ducts than in the lobules. It may be helpful to know a few technical terms:

- **Ductal carcinoma in situ (DCIS)** means the cancer is contained within the duct and has not spread farther. It's noninvasive and generally doesn't have the ability to spread. We call it stage 0 cancer.
- **Invasive ductal or lobular carcinoma (IDC or ILC)** means the cancer has spread outside the duct or lobule. It can be stage I through IV. The difference between invasive ductal carcinoma and invasive lobular carcinoma is where in the breast the cancer originated. The pathologist who looks at the slides from your biopsy will determine which type of cancer it is. Sometimes breast cancer has features of both ductal and lobular carcinomas; this type of cancer is called invasive mammary carcinoma. It's not necessarily the case that the cancer originated in both the duct and the lobules. Rather, it may have features of both. It doesn't change prognosis or stage—it's just a pathologic description of the kinds of cells the cancer originated from.
- **Lobular carcinoma in situ (LCIS)** is another type of pathology. Although it has the word "carcinoma" in it, it's *not* a cancer, but having LCIS substantially increases your lifetime risk of breast cancer. However, since it's *not* cancer, it isn't discussed in this chapter; we'll cover it in chapter 5, which addresses conditions that increase your risk of breast cancer.

LYMPH NODES

The lymphatic system is the body's filtration system. Lymph nodes filter the lymphatic fluid, which carries waste products and destroyed bacteria back into the bloodstream; the liver or kidneys then remove these from the blood. Lymphatics also maintain fluid levels in our body and are part of the process of removing debris like dead cells and cancer cells. The lymph nodes in the axilla (armpit) manage fluid that drains from the arm and the breast. They might become enlarged after a vaccine shot because of the inflammation that occurs, but can also become enlarged due to involvement by cancer.

The thing that's fascinating is that lymphatic drainage is a very organized system. There are hundreds, perhaps even thousands, of lymph nodes throughout the body, and every part of the body has designated lymph nodes that drain that specific part. These lymph nodes are all connected by very small tubes known as the lymphatics or lymph vessels. When one part of the body is drained by the lymphatics, the first lymph node gets the drainage first, then the second node, and so on. Think of it as a railway system. The lymphatic system is the tracks and nodes are the train stations. When the train leaves the station, it goes in an orderly way to each subsequent station. That's what happens with the lymphatics and the lymph nodes. It's why when you have a cold, the lymph nodes in your neck may temporarily get larger— they're filtering the infection.

Whenever there's an invasive breast cancer, we need to determine if the cancer has spread beyond the breast to the lymph nodes, since this will impact the stage of diagnosis as well as what kind of treatment is needed. Since the breast drains to the lymph nodes in the armpit in an organized way, we check the first node, and if that's negative, we can safely assume that the rest of the nodes are as well. The first draining node is called the sentinel lymph node. It's the guarding node, essentially protecting the rest of the nodes. If the sentinel lymph nodes don't have cancer, it's safe to assume that the other nodes in your armpits, or axillae, don't have cancer. Many women have more than one sentinel lymph node, since the breast may drain to more than one group of nodes. Your surgeon may discuss doing a sentinel node biopsy at the time of surgery. The sentinel node is identified by the injection of a compound—often a blue dye, a low-dose radioactive compound, or both—into the breast; then when the compound drains from the breast, the surgeon can identify which lymph node it drains into. This process should identify all the sentinel nodes in the breast. How many lymph nodes you have removed will be determined at the time of surgery. If there's cancer in the sentinel lymph nodes, then more lymph nodes may need to be removed (a procedure known as axillary lymph node dissection) to determine how many lymph nodes are involved with cancer. This number will likely impact your doctor's recommendations for what kind of treatments you will need.

Your lymph nodes may initially be evaluated by radiologists with imaging, such as ultrasound or MRI, to see if they're enlarged. To find out whether there are cancer cells in the lymph nodes, a needle biopsy may be recommended before surgery so the pathologist can examine the lymph node. Although imaging can strongly suggest if a lymph node is involved with cancer by the size, shape, and characteristics of that node, the definitive determination is made when the lymph node that was removed is examined by the pathologist, both at the time of surgery and in more detail afterward.

STAGE AND GRADE

"Grade" refers to how cancer cells look under the microscope when the pathologist examines the tissue, and how much they're dividing. Tumor grades range from 1 to 3, with 3 being the most aggressive. Sometimes it's helpful to think of grade as how different the breast cancer cell is from a normal breast cell. The cancer cell that looks most similar to a normal breast cell is grade 1, and the one that looks the most different from a normal breast cell is grade 3. Of course, a grade 2 cancer cell is between.

"Stage" refers to an overall assessment of the cancer. The stage is determined by the size of the tumor, the involvement of lymph nodes, and the spread of the tumor to other parts of the body. This is different from the grade of the tumor. The stage of the cancer is used to determine survival statistics and whether chemotherapy is needed, as well as other factors.

- **Stage I:** The tumor measures two centimeters or less, and the lymph nodes are negative or have micrometastases (microscopic tumors in which less than two millimeters of the lymph node are involved with the cancer cells).
- **Stage II:** The tumor measures more than two centimeters, or there's involvement of fewer than four lymph nodes.
- **Stage III:** The tumor measures more than five centimeters (with positive lymph nodes) or involves skin, or there are four or more lymph nodes involved.
- **Stage IV:** The cancer has spread beyond the breast and the lymph nodes that drain it; the cancer has spread to other organs or to the bones.

TREATMENT

The best treatment for you will be based on the biology of your particular cancer.

In the past, the standard protocol was to do surgery first; then chemotherapy, if necessary; then radiation, if a lumpectomy was performed. Thanks to many studies, we now know that different types of cancer benefit from different types of treatment, and sometimes even from a particular sequence or order of treatments, to afford more personalized and effective care.

There are many different types of breast cancer. To determine what type of breast cancer you have, pathologists test for three receptors: estrogen, progesterone, and HER2/neu. The main subtypes of tumors are:

- **Luminal A/Luminal B** (50 to 60 percent). Slow-growing tumors that respond well to hormone suppression or endocrine therapy, but are often not responsive to chemotherapy.
- **HER2 positive** (20 percent). Fast-growing tumors with extra copies of the gene that makes HER2 proteins. The targeted cancer drug Herceptin (trastuzumab; see page 52) is highly effective at targeting and killing breast cancer cells with HER2 receptors.
- **Triple-negative** (15 to 20 percent). Fast-growing tumors; called "triple-negative" because the breast cancer cells have no estrogen, no progesterone, and no HER2 receptors on their surface. Most hereditary breast cancers are triple-negative. Often responds well to chemotherapy, and may respond well to targeted immunotherapy.

Hormone-Positive Tumors

Luminal A/luminal B tumors cancers start in the duct (lumen) of the breast and have estrogen and/or progesterone receptors on their surface, which they need for growth. Think of estrogen and progesterone like fuel for a fire: Without the fuel, the fire will stop growing. Similarly, if you suppress estrogen and/or progesterone, the tumor stops growing.

- **Luminal A tumors** are slow-growing tumors that respond well to hormone suppression; they have the best prognosis and the lowest rate of recurrence. They don't have HER2 receptors on their surface, and typically are not affected by chemotherapy, so chemotherapy is generally not used or needed to improve survival outlooks. This type of breast cancer is treated with hormonal therapy.

- **Luminal B tumors** are also hormone responsive, but have a more rapid tumor growth and a higher grade (the way the cancer cells look under the microscope) than luminal A tumors. The cancer cells may have HER2 receptors on their surface. Luminal B cancers are more often diagnosed in younger women and are always treated with hormonal therapy.
- **Luminal A/B tumors** both respond to hormonal therapy, in which estrogen and/or progesterone is suppressed. Some luminal A/B tumors benefit from chemotherapy. The best way to tell is with genomic testing.

GENOMIC TESTING

Genomic testing has been a game changer. It specifically tests *your* tumor to determine whether it will respond to chemotherapy; if it won't, chemotherapy will not be recommended, because there would be no significant improvement in survival with chemotherapy. There are a number of different types of genomic testing. They all test a significant number of the genes your tumor has and, based on that, can let us know if it would be helpful to add chemotherapy to your treatment plan. Examining your tumor to best develop a treatment plan specifically for you is truly personalized medicine. It allows us to provide risk of recurrence of the tumor for early-stage cancers so we can give each patient a personal treatment plan tailored to their needs.

The two most common genomic tests are Oncotype DX and MammaPrint. In the US, Oncotype DX is the most common genomic test used; in parts of Europe, MammaPrint is used more frequently.

Oncotype DX is a twenty-one-gene expression assay done for breast cancers that are ER-positive HER2-negative tumors to help determine if chemotherapy is necessary. The test is ordered after either a needle biopsy or, more often, after surgery. Once some or all of the cancerous tissue has been removed, part of the cancer is sent to a lab that evaluates twenty-one different genes on the tumor and gives information about the tumor's biology, reporting scores that range from 0 to 100. A score of less than 18 is considered to be low for premenopausal women; for postmenopausal women, less than 25 is low. When the score is low, it means that the tumor is low risk for recurrence and giving chemotherapy won't help (and therefore, we don't). We recommend genomic testing for patients who are premenopausal with negative lymph nodes, and those who are postmenopausal with negative lymph nodes or with one to three positive lymph nodes. If there are more than three lymph nodes involved in postmenopausal women, or any lymph nodes involved in women who are premenopausal, then chemotherapy is recommended, since we worry about the tumor recurring. The tumor is high risk by virtue of how far it has extended at the time of diagnosis, and high-risk breast cancer is essentially always treated with chemotherapy.

MammaPrint, another type of genomic testing, is used less frequently in the US but more frequently in Europe. Unlike Oncotype DX, it can also be used on triple-negative cancers to determine if chemotherapy is needed. MammaPrint tests seventy genes and is used in some practices to evaluate both hormone-receptor-positive and hormone-receptor-negative breast cancers. This is a lot of information, and quite specific, but it's information that you need to determine your best path forward.

Genomic testing can be used before surgery to determine if drugs such as tamoxifen or aromatase inhibitors, both of which block estrogen's effects on cancers, should be used first to try to shrink a large tumor to make it more amenable to surgery. If the score is low, chemotherapy wouldn't be effective and therefore isn't used. Adding chemotherapy would only be detrimental in this instance; it won't help treat the cancer, and you will still have to cope with the side effects of chemotherapy.

Definitive studies have shown that the outcome for women with low genomic scores won't change even if chemotherapy is given. Conversely, studies have shown that for women whose scores are high, chemotherapy would be effective. If the score is intermediate, multiple other factors, including the patient's personal preference, are used to decide if chemotherapy is given. These issues should be part of the discussion between you and your oncologist.

HORMONAL THERAPY

The therapy for luminal A/B cancers involves blocking estrogen and/or progesterone from attaching to these cancer cells. So, actually, it's antiestrogen or antihormone therapy—the opposite of hormone replacement therapy (HRT). It's also called endocrine therapy. Antiestrogen therapy works against hormone-receptor-positive breast cancer. For women diagnosed with ER-positive cancers, some oncologists may recommend avoiding diets high in soy products, since soy contains phytoestrogens (natural estrogens derived from plants). Studies have shown that consuming natural soy products is safe and may even be beneficial. We don't recommend eliminating phytoestrogens altogether, but moderation is best.

Tamoxifen is the most commonly used hormone therapy drug. It has been used for over forty years to treat ER-positive early, locally advanced, and metastatic breast cancers. It's a selective estrogen receptor modulator (SERM) that attaches to the hormone receptors in the cancer cell and blocks estrogen from attaching, preventing the cells from growing. It's the drug of choice for:

- **Premenopausal women** diagnosed with breast cancer.
- **Postmenopausal women** who have osteoporosis, as it has some protective effect on the bones.

- **Risk reduction** in patients who do not have cancer but are at increased risk for breast cancer, such as women who have had a breast biopsy that has shown atypical ductal hyperplasia (ADH) or lobular carcinoma in situ (LCIS), or who have a strong family history of breast cancer.

Tamoxifen is taken daily for five to ten years. As with all drugs, there are side effects. The most common side effects of tamoxifen are hot flashes and vaginal discharge. However, tamoxifen may cause an increased risk of uterine cancer and blood clots, and cannot be used in patients who are at increased risk for blood clots.

Aromatase inhibitors stop the production of estrogen by blocking aromatase, an enzyme that converts hormones called androgens into estrogen. The three main aromatase inhibitors are

- Anastrozole (Arimidex)
- Exemestane (Aromasin)
- Letrozole (Femara)

These are the medications of choice in postmenopausal women with hormone-receptor-positive breast cancer, since premenopausal women's ovaries make too much estrogen to have signficant effects from aromatase inhibitors. Aromatase inhibitors can be used only in premenopausal women whose ovarian function is suppressed, since the amount of estrogen made by the ovaries overwhelms the effect of aromatase inhibitors. Ovarian function in premenopausal women can be suppressed with drugs such as Lupron and Zoladex.

The suppression of ovarian function reduces the amount of estrogen in the body, so there's less estrogen to stimulate the growth of hormone-receptor-positive breast cancer cells. If a premenopausal woman has advanced breast cancer with positive lymph nodes, her ovarian function can be stopped by either surgically removing the ovaries or using drugs to stop their functioning so that an aromatase inhibitor can be used. In the latter case, ovarian function may return after the drugs are stopped following treatment for breast cancer. However, this isn't always the case and depends on many factors, including the age of the woman at the time of treatment, with older women less likely to have return of their ovarian function after treatment, the type of drugs that were used for treatment, or both.

Aromatase inhibitors are generally taken daily for five to ten years. Side effects can include joint stiffness or pain and increased risk for bone loss, resulting in osteoporosis or osteopenia.

Chemotherapy is recommended if there's a high genomic score in ER/PR-positive breast cancer, indicating a high-risk cancer, which requires chemotherapy for optimal treatment, or if there are positive lymph nodes. Two different chemotherapeutic regimens are recommended.

- **For node-negative premenopausal women and older women,** Taxol (paclitaxel) and Cytoxan (cyclophosphamide) are administered every three weeks for four cycles. These drugs are generally tolerated very well and can often be given intravenously in the arm without a Mediport (see below).
- **Women with positive lymph nodes and higher-risk cancer** generally receive dose-dense chemotherapy; this is also the type of chemotherapy given to women with triple-negative breast cancer (see page 45), since that's intrinsically a high-risk cancer and is always treated with chemotherapy. It requires a Mediport.

MEDIPORT
A Mediport is a small piece of plastic with a membrane into which needles can be inserted accurately and with minimal discomfort.

It makes giving chemotherapy safer and reduces the number of "sticks" needed to get access to veins. Chemotherapy can be very harmful to the arm veins because it's a caustic chemical. Placement of a Mediport is done by a surgeon or an interventional radiologist. Sedation and anesthesia are used during the procedure. A catheter is placed in a vein in the neck and attached to a port, which is placed under the skin. There will be a one-inch incision in the upper chest area where the port is placed, and a quarter-inch incision in the neck where the catheter is placed. In thinner women, the port can be visible as a bulge in the skin. Once it has healed, most normal activities can be resumed; extremely vigorous activities may be discouraged. When you've completed chemotherapy, the Mediport can be removed.

The advantage of a Mediport is that it can be used not only to deliver chemotherapy but also for taking blood draws and delivering intravenous fluids if they're necessary. Before each appointment, you will be given topical numbing medication to put on the skin overlying the port. Your nurse will then access the port with a Huber needle, which is generally not painful.

For HER2-Positive Tumors

About 20 percent of breast cancer tumors are HER2 positive. HER2 is the abbreviated name for human epidermal growth factor receptor-2. Compared to other cancers, these tumors tend to grow quickly and are more likely to spread. The good news is that they're very responsive to targeted therapy. Targeted therapy using a drug such as Herceptin specifically binds to the HER2 receptor on the surface of breast cancer cells, preventing HER2 from attaching to the cells. Since the cancer cells need this protein to grow, blocking the receptors means that cell growth is blocked as well.

Targeted therapy for HER2-positive breast cancers works differently than chemotherapy. It's given intravenously, but it usually has fewer side effects than chemotherapy. A number of drugs have been developed to target HER2 cells; they're all highly effective. A Mediport will be recommended for HER2-positive breast cancer treatment.

MONOCLONAL ANTIBODIES FOR HER2-POSITIVE BREAST CANCER

Monoclonal antibodies are the most common type of targeted therapy. They're man-made immune system proteins that attach to the HER2 protein on cancer cells to stop the cells from growing. The cells need HER2 to grow. Think of the cells' HER2 receptors as a lock and HER2 as the matching key. In order for the cells to grow, you need to unlock the lock with the perfectly fitting key. Targeted therapy is essentially a specific "plug" that sits in the lock, preventing the key from entering and thereby preventing the cells from growing. It's targeted because, as every lock has a specific key that fits perfectly to unlock it, so too the protein has to fit perfectly in the lock. HER2 is the perfectly fitting key that unlocks the cells' ability to grow, and the monoclonal antibodies are the perfectly fitting plug that prohibits HER2 from unlocking the cells' ability to grow. The drugs are not chemotherapy, which kills healthy cells as well as cancerous ones, and, as such, targeted therapy generally doesn't have the negative side effects of chemotherapy.

- **Herceptin** (trastuzumab) is most commonly used for both early-stage and advanced cancers. It's given initially with chemotherapy, and then every three weeks for a year after chemotherapy is complete. Side effects include headache, diarrhea, nausea, and chills. The most concerning, but rare, side effects of Herceptin are problems with heart function, so you will have an echocardiogram before and often after treatment. During treatment, if you develop shortness of breath, swelling of the ankles, or a weight gain of five pounds or more in twenty-four hours, contact your doctor. Your medical oncologist will monitor your echocardiogram and symptoms and, if necessary, refer you to a cardiologist.

- **Perjeta** (pertuzumab) is commonly given with Herceptin (transtuzumab) for women with advanced cancers that are larger than two centimeters, those who have positive lymph nodes, and those who have metastatic breast cancer. When Perjeta is given with Herceptin and chemotherapy, it can cause significant diarrhea.

- **Phesgo**, a combination of Herceptin (transtuzumab) and Perjeta (pertuzumab), can be given subcutaneously (injected under the skin), not intravenously. Therefore, the Mediport can be removed once chemotherapy is over, rather than giving Herceptin and Perjeta intravenously for a year.

- **Kadcyla** (trastuzumab emtansine) is a combination of Herceptin and chemotherapy. It provides both HER2-targeted treatment and chemotherapy at the same time, with fewer side effects of chemotherapy. Treatment with Herceptin and chemotherapy is most often given before surgery, but may be given after breast cancer surgery for early-stage cancers.

Early-stage HER2-positive breast cancers that are small (less than two centimeters, or about three-quarters of an inch) and when lymph nodes are not involved are generally treated with surgery first. This gives information to the medical oncologist about whether a less aggressive chemotherapy can be given with Herceptin since the tumor itself is needed to determine response to the drugs. If the final pathology confirms that the tumor is less than two centimeters and the lymph nodes are negative, the recommended regimen is Herceptin with the chemotherapy drug

Taxol (paclitaxel) weekly for a total of twelve cycles, or three months. Side effects, which don't happen to everyone, may include neuropathy (tingling and numbness in the fingers and toes), fatigue, and low white blood cell count.

For patients with HER2-positive tumors larger than two centimeters who have positive lymph nodes or locally advanced cancers, neoadjuvant treatment (treatment before surgery) with Herceptin and Perjeta along with chemotherapy is recommended. Studies have shown that giving the chemotherapy before surgery can show if the tumor is responding and, in fact, result in better outcomes for the patient. The chemotherapy drugs given include Taxotere (docetaxel) and carboplatin. This regimen is given once every three weeks for six cycles, so eighteen weeks in total. In addition to the aforementioned diarrhea, side effects (which, again, don't occur in every person) include hair loss, fatigue, muscle and joint aches, heartburn, nausea, and nail changes. Many medications, both over-the-counter or prescribed by your doctor, are available to improve symptoms of nausea and diarrhea.

Once chemotherapy is complete, Herceptin with or without Perjeta will be continued every three weeks for a year. If residual cancer is seen after surgery for patients treated with neoadjuvant chemotherapy, Kadcyla will be recommended. Hormonal therapy may be given in addition to the chemotherapy and targeted for ER/PR-positive cancer. If you're going to receive radiation, it will be given during the time that Herceptin and Perjeta are given.

The chemotherapeutic regimens described here are the ones that, at present, are most frequently used. These regimens can change, and therefore, the exact course of treatment you get will be determined after extensive discussion with your medical oncologist and will be based on the latest available data concerning the most effective therapies.

Triple-Negative Tumors

Triple-negative breast cancers don't have estrogen, progesterone, or HER2 receptors on their cell surface. They're an aggressive type of breast cancer and therefore almost always require chemotherapy.

Chemotherapy occurs before surgery (unless the tumor is less than one centimeter) in a dose-dense AC-T regimen: Adriamycin (doxorubicin) and Cytoxan (cyclophosphamide) every two weeks for four cycles, then Taxol (paclitaxel) every two weeks for four cycles. Neoadjuvant immunotherapy (Keytruda) along with chemotherapy is now also being offered in clinical trials.

Women with triple-negative breast cancer often show an excellent response to neoadjuvant chemotherapy (chemotherapy before surgery). Even if imaging shows no more cancer present after the neoadjuvant chemotherapy, they still need surgery, as there may be remaining cancer cells that are too small to see with imaging. If residual cancer is found, additional therapy with a chemotherapy pill called Xeloda (capecitabine) might be recommended.

Side effects for both Adriamycin and Taxol include nausea, diarrhea, vomiting, joint pain, flushing, dizziness, and drowsiness; neuropathy is more likely to occur with Taxol than Adriamycin. Adriamycin may cause heart damage, so an echocardiogram will be performed before and after treatment. Cytoxan can cause severe nausea and vomiting, so drugs may be prescribed to reduce these symptoms. All three drugs cause hair loss. For patients receiving Taxol, cold caps (see page 59) are an option to decrease or avoid loss of hair. Cold caps are exactly what they sound like: ice or cold caps placed on the head during and for a time after chemotherapy. The cold causes the blood vessels in the scalp to constrict, decreasing blood flow and limiting the amount of chemotherapy that goes to the scalp. Unfortunately, cold caps don't work well with dose-dense chemotherapy.

GENETIC TESTING

All patients with triple-negative breast cancer should have the opportunity to undergo genetic testing to see if they may have a gene that significantly increases their risk of breast cancer, like the BRCA gene. A positive genetic test may warrant the addition of carboplatin (Paraplatin) to Taxol in the second half of treatment. More recent studies have demonstrated that the addition of carboplatin is very effective in treating cancers in women who have these genetic mutations, and the cancers that occur in these women are types that respond well to platinum-based therapy. If that's necessary, treatment with carboplatin will last three weeks for six cycles. The side effects are similar to those described for Taxol on page 54, but more severe fatigue and nausea may occur.

Many studies are being conducted to determine whether genomic profiling might optimize care with different chemotherapy regimens. There are many clinical trials evaluating Xeloda, immunotherapy, PARP inhibitors, and other targeted therapies for patients with recurrent or advanced disease and for those with a genetic predisposition to breast cancer. It's a rapidly changing landscape and provides much hope for the future.

Metastatic Breast Cancer

Metastatic breast cancer, although not curable and with generally lower survival rates, may be successfully managed for many years and may be thought of as a chronic disease like high blood pressure or diabetes, diseases which are not cured but may be successfully managed for many years. Women with metastatic breast cancer have cancer beyond their breasts, and therefore, removing the breasts, or mastectomy, may not help, since it doesn't eradicate the cancer.

Treatments for women with metastatic breast cancer will have to be varied to adapt to the individual situation. They may start on a drug regimen that the tumor responds well to only to find that after some time, the cancer continues to grow, what we call "breaking through" the treatment. When this happens, the patient's regimen is changed to expose the cancer to a drug that may be newly effective. This new drug regimen is effective for some time, but it may be that the cancer finds a way around the drug, and the regimen needs to change again.

It's important to know that there are many treatment options for breast cancer, and more are being discovered every day. These new and more effective approaches to treating breast cancer are found through clinical trials. Clinical trials are critical to finding new methods of treatment and new drugs to treat breast cancer. Therefore, if you're offered the opportunity to participate in a clinical trial, it's important to seriously consider it. Not only could the newer approaches be more effective for your cancer (although you won't know that to be true until after the trial is complete), these trials are the only way to scientifically and rigorously evaluate new treatments for breast cancer. By participating, you may benefit not only yourself but countless others as well. Women of color have historically been underrepresented in clinical trials, and it's important that this misrepresentation be corrected. To achieve the optimal therapy for different types of cancers, women of all races must participate in clinical trials so we can learn all we can about new treatments—not only if they work but in what population they work best (or don't work).

Trying to find information online can be helpful, as can advice from friends (sometimes helpful but generally not, since every person's breast cancer, pathologies, biology, and response to various therapies will be different). Therefore, a word of caution here: Many people in your life will want to share their breast cancer experiences with you, but be wary, since every situation and every breast cancer is different, and your treatment, your response to your treatment, and your possible side effects may be very different too. In general, conversations with your physician and, if necessary, a second opinion from another physician will be the most successful way to determine the best treatment for you.

Radiation

The treatment for breast cancer is either mastectomy or partial mastectomy (lumpectomy) and radiation. Most women who undergo a partial mastectomy need radiation to ensure that no additional cancer cells are lurking in the nearby tissue. Even women who have had a mastectomy may require radiation if their lymph nodes were involved with cancer. If even one lymph node is involved, women with triple-negative cancers can increase their chances of survival by having radiation. Radiation may be also recommended after a mastectomy if the original tumor measured more than five centimeters, or if the surrounding area was involved.

RADIATION REGIMEN

With a few exceptions, women who have had their breast cancer treated with breast conservation, also referred to as partial mastectomy or lumpectomy, will require radiation therapy. Typical radiation therapy will involve treatment every weekday—Monday through Friday—for four to six weeks. The treatments are not painful, and last about ten minutes.

Side effects may include skin redness and pain as well as fatigue. In the long term, radiation may cause a hardening of the breast, especially if tissue was used for reconstruction and if an implant is present. The skin on the breast may feel noticeably tighter after radiation therapy.

In recent years, shorter radiation therapy regimens have been developed. In some cases, one dose of intraoperative radiation is sufficient, but the number of women who are candidates for this option are limited. Another option is partial breast radiation, which is completed in five days. The type of radiation you receive will depend on many factors, which is why this decision will be made by you and your radiation oncologist if even one lymph node is involved. New options are constantly being developed, so be sure to talk to your radiation oncologist about the possibilities and best treatment for you.

Tips for Side Effects

Over the years, our patients have passed along wonderful tips that can help ameliorate some of the unpleasant side effects of these lifesaving treatments. Along with the tips here, you can find many more in cancer therapy chat rooms and social media groups online. But remember, some of these suggestions, like cold caps, are based on solid scientific data, and some are not. Even those that are more anecdotal may be worth a try—they may well help—but again, a caution that much on the internet is not scientifically based, or even proven in any way. Some of the things on the internet can actually be harmful; therefore, always ask a member of your care team for advice. Your care team is there for you!

- **For nail issues:** Almost half (44 percent) of patients experience changes in their nails, the worst of which is nail loss. Others experience alteration of the nail, such as darkening. Applying nail polish can help cover any discoloration.[1] A topical herbal balm may significantly reduce nail damage.[2]
- **For neuropathy:** Wearing cold gloves and socks (cryotherapy) was shown to reduce neuropathy (tingling and numbness in the fingers/toes) and nail changes in a significant number of patients in a small study.[3]
- **For hair loss:** To reduce hair loss, cold caps can be used. Cold caps are ice-cold caps worn on your head before, during, and for two hours after chemotherapy. The cold narrows the blood

vessels to the scalp, thereby reducing blood flow and, as a result, the amount of chemotherapy drug that reaches the hair follicles. This results in less of the effects of chemotherapy on those cells, reducing hair loss. Cold caps are not equally effective with different chemotherapies. With some, they work well, and hair is preserved. With others, the chemotherapy will lead to hair loss even with cold capping. Cold capping works best with Taxol (paclitaxel) or Taxotere (docetaxel) chemotherapy.

Some women have success with these options. Others find the drawbacks too challenging. When cold caps work, for instance, women still lose about half their hair. Side effects include chills, headaches, neck and shoulder discomfort, and scalp pain. The caps must be tightly fitted, which can make them uncomfortable. Women undergoing cold cap treatment can only wash their hair once a week. Initially, insurance generally didn't cover cold cap treatments, since it was considered cosmetic. Some insurance companies now do provide coverage, and hopefully all will soon—they should. We feel that there should be a law requiring that cold cap therapy be covered, should the patient choose it. Many women and men feel that hair loss signals to the world around them that they're cancer patients, and that for months after chemotherapy is complete, hair loss remains a constant reminder of their cancer therapy. For some people, until their hair has grown back, they aren't done with treatment. That's why we feel so strongly that insurance should cover the cost of cold capping. If you would like to give cold capping a try, the most common systems, DigniCap and Paxman scalp cooling systems, are now approved by the FDA and supported by solid scientific data.

One of our patients, Liz Lord, absolutely dreaded the thought of losing her hair from chemotherapy. This was before we instituted one of the country's first cold cap programs at the George Washington University Hospital. Cold capping helped Liz keep half her hair; she was so happy that she not only helped educate our nurses about the importance of cold capping, she started a foundation called Cold Capital Fund (coldcapitalfund.org) to fund cold caps for women in Virginia, Maryland, and Washington, DC, who cannot afford them. One of the silver linings of breast cancer treatment is how some who have gone through this experience, like Liz, find ways to use it to help others. There may be a similar foundation to help cover the cost of cold capping in your area. Don't hesitate to ask or to reach out to Cold Capital Fund. They may be able to help you.

RECOVERY
Complementary and Integrative Medicine

Complementary and integrative medicine (CIM) combines conventional treatments with alternative medicines and modalities. We certainly don't recommend following an exclusively alternative medicinal approach—in fact, we strongly caution against it. Conventional therapy is based on science and rigorous clinical studies, and not all alternative medicine is supported by rigorous science. It's also true that many alternative therapies, even though not supported by research and data, are not harmful and may be helpful to some—but only when they're used in conjunction with conventional therapy.

Patients who are eager to try alternative treatments alone as their initial treatment may not realize that while they're exploring potential treatments, their condition may be getting worse. We've seen women delay conventional, scientifically supported treatments while exploring or undergoing alternative therapies only to return to us when the disease has significantly progressed and their prognosis is worse. We discourage all women from avoiding conventional therapy. The results can be deadly.

CIM takes a holistic approach to treating patients and combines conventional oncologic treatments with alternative modalities for maximal healing effects. It doesn't dismiss conventional medicine but combines treatments to relieve symptoms and ease side effects. CIM is based on the presumption that healing is unique for each patient. Some complementary medicinal modalities are supported by research and are medically safe. Some are not, but may still be helpful, and may be recommended when they're not harmful. In our practice, we've found that CIM can be a beneficial way to guide patients to mental and physical wellness as they go through conventional treatments.

Christy came to support complementary medicine after the experience of her best friend, Laurie. At thirty-four years old, Laurie was diagnosed with breast cancer. Laurie was living in Colorado, and at the time, unlike many places in the United States, CIM was not only recognized as an integral component to therapy for patients in Colorado, medical insurance covered it. When Laurie met with a naturopathic doctor, she learned about herbal therapies that might reduce symptoms from chemotherapy. Later she used acupuncture to reduce her side effects from surgery and chemotherapy, as well as Reiki and yoga to help her get through the stresses of cancer treatment. However, Laurie also had conventional scientifically based therapy during her course of treatment.

CIM is recommended for those who feel they would benefit from it. Rachel chose not to pursue CIM during her treatment, as she felt that the available conventional approaches worked for her. That said, we feel that it's an option that should be considered and available to all who are interested. At George Washington University, we now have an excellent Center for Integrative Medicine and have many shared programs that benefit our patients as they go through treatment. We provide services to our patients through fundraising to support our Patient Assistance

Fund. Therefore, even when not covered by insurance and not affordable to some of our patients, all can have CIM as part of their treatment. More and more breast centers are now offering such services. Our ultimate goal is that insurance will cover treatments so that all women in all centers who wish to have access to CIM can. Although we support CIM, we believe that every woman should pursue the path that's best for her, as long as she *always* receives conventional, scientifically based therapy.

Naturopathic Medicine

A comprehensive approach to healing that combines traditional and natural forms of medicine is offered by naturopaths (NDs), who have trained at accredited four-year naturopathic medical schools. Naturopathy includes both the study of conventional medical sciences and a broad range of natural and noninvasive therapies, including nutrition, herbal therapy, homeopathy, lifestyle counseling, and physical medicine. Many NDs are also trained in acupuncture, which has been shown in many studies to benefit patients undergoing chemotherapy and even those experiencing hot flashes. Combining the cutting-edge treatments created by the latest science with ancient life-enhancing remedies that have helped for thousands of years gives us the best of both worlds. A positive attitude and optimal medical therapy, along with CIM for those who want it, will be the best path to achieving your best treatment and outcome. Therefore, while your care team should always include medical and surgical oncologists, it may also include naturopaths to help with the side effects and physical and emotional impact of cancer and its conventional treatment. Naturopaths alone should not be directing your cancer care.

Nutritional counseling can be provided by an ND or a registered dietician. Visits with an ND are considered complementary medicine and therefore are likely not covered by insurance. However, most centers have a dietician on site who will be able to give counseling about diet recommendations during treatments if it's necessary, as well as for weight loss or weight gain for those who need it. Visits with dieticians are covered by the various centers and are of no cost to patients. Christy has a special interest in nutrition since it was her major in college, and often makes recommendations to patients about both nutrition and exercise.

Acupuncture
Originating in China around 6000 BCE, this treatment, in which very thin needles are placed along the natural lines of energy in the body, has proven itself over millennia. Studies have shown that acupuncture can reduce nausea and vomiting as well as other side effects from chemotherapy. Other benefits include managing pain, hot flashes, peripheral neuropathy, joint pain, and other side effects from chemotherapy and/or radiation therapy. Ongoing acupuncture treatments are completely safe and well tolerated by most patients.

Most states requiring specific licensing for providers who perform acupuncture. Many NDs are licensed to perform acupuncture. Many major cancer centers across the country have had acupuncture incorporated into their cancer care for more than a decade, including George Washington University, Dana-Farber Cancer Institute, Memorial Sloan Kettering Cancer Center, and MD Anderson Cancer Center.[4] Again, this is in addition to the necessary care by your oncologists (medical and surgical) to optimally treat your breast cancer.

Yoga
Yoga, too, has been around since antiquity. The movements and poses that have been perfected over centuries have been bene-

ficial to people undergoing treatment for cancer. Research has long shown that a skilled practitioner of yoga can control their physical functions, such as blood pressure, heart rate, breathing, metabolism, body temperature, brain waves, and skin resistance. This can result in improved physical fitness, lower levels of stress, and increased feelings of relaxation and well-being. Those who practice yoga may also have less stress and fatigue and a better quality of life. However, like everything during your treatment, ask your doctor if yoga is right for you.

Reiki

This technique is performed by a practitioner to create energy balance and healing, promote relaxation, and reduce anxiety. Studies show that it's useful for pain and anxiety.[5] Some of our patients find Reiki helps them relax before surgery, chemotherapy, or other necessary treatments. Some don't. See what works for you.

Massage Therapy

Patients often find that massage gives them welcome relief from cancer treatments and may help them avoid narcotics, speed healing, and facilitate a body-mind-spirit balance. Massage can help patients restore their baseline function as quickly as possible and relieve pain and stress. Many of us love getting massages in our regular lives, but after surgery, it can be important for recovery. Be sure to ask your doctor before making an appointment; massage isn't always recommended during chemotherapy and other therapies.

Physical Therapy

Physical therapists (PTs) can help with the physical symptoms of breast cancer and its treatment. They use scientifically based techniques to help reduce pain and discomfort of the musculoskeletal system. The exercises they offer can help alleviate symptoms far more quickly than is possible without physical therapy.

After mastectomy, physical therapy is frequently used to improve the mobility of the arm, particularly after lymph node dissection. After implant or expander reconstructions, the chest and back muscles are often very tight. PTs can help loosen these muscles and return them to normal again. This may help speed up your recovery by several weeks.

Many PTs specialize in lymphedema education and management. Lymphedema is a swelling of the arm after lymphatic damage caused by lymph node dissection. The swelling is a result of normal lymph fluid drainage that can be worsened when there is an infection in the arm, after excessive activity, or because of pressure changes, such as those encountered during air travel. When your doctor knows beforehand that a lymph node dissection will be necessary, she will often refer you to a PT specialist for baseline measurements before surgery and treatment afterward. If the referral is made after surgery, it's fine. The important thing is that you receive the valuable treatment and education from the PT about how best to avoid lymphedema. However, even with physical therapy and taking all the precautions, some women may develop lymphedema. Lymphedema occurs in up to 25 percent of women who have full axillary lymph node dissections for breast cancer due to cancer involvement of the nodes. You should know that if you develop lymphedema, it isn't anything you did but how your body responded to the surgery you had. If you do develop it, your dedicated physical therapist can help you manage your symptoms and minimize swelling in your arms. We recommend that you develop a relationship with a PT and decide what is best for you.

For many women, lymphedema therapy is ongoing, even lifelong. There's really no way to absolutely prevent lymphedema. It's best to develop a relationship with your PT to try to minimize significant lymphedema.

Christy's friend Laurie provides an example of this. On a visit to Washington, DC, one winter, she was helping shovel snow from the driveway. Afterward, the arm in which she had had a lymph node dissection years before was swollen. Her flight to DC and shoveling snow had caused mild lymphedema. We wrapped her arm in Ace bandages to reduce swelling, and when she got home, she met with her physical therapist for lymphatic drainage. Because she caught it early, she has not had a problem since. For some women, even if you treat lymphedema early, it isn't always curable, but it *is* always treatable. However, it's important to realize that even with treatment there may well be a difference in the size of your arms, with the side after lymph node dissection remaining larger throughout your life.

OVERVIEW

The field of breast cancer is dynamic, and research is constantly changing diagnosis and treatment options for patients. The therapy is becoming more personalized and based on the molecular profile of your cancer. Always ask your doctor about the newest therapies available and any promising ones that are still in development or in clinical trials.

Keep in mind that the prognosis for breast cancer has improved dramatically over the past two decades. The death rate from breast cancer has decreased by over 40 percent since the late 1980s, a remarkable accomplishment owing to improved screening, earlier detection, and improved therapies.

Even patients who have metastatic disease can enjoy life far longer than ever before. Today, there's good reason to hope that even those with recurrent or metastatic cancer have hope for prolonged survival. In fact, there's an increasing trend to think of some metastatic breast cancers as a chronic disease, much like hypertension or diabetes: we can't cure the disease, but many can live long, productive, and fulfilling lives with it.

This chapter has a lot of information about different areas of breast cancer treatment. Every single person with breast cancer is different, and there are numerous types of breast cancer. Be sure to have extensive discussions with your care team about all aspects of breast cancer—and never hesitate to ask them any question that's on your mind. It's not only your right—it's your responsibility. Most of all, we wish you the best and hope for the best for you and your loved ones.

Common Questions to Discuss with Your Care Team

Where exactly in my breast(s) do I have cancer?

What does it mean if it's a ductal or lobular cancer?

What does the grade mean?

What stage is the cancer?

What are my receptors, and what does that mean for my treatment?

What is my risk for recurrence?

What is my expected survival?

Should I get genetic testing?

Can you explain my pathology report to me?

What are my treatment options?

When will I meet with a medical oncologist?

When should I meet with a radiation oncologist?

Do I have the option of having mastectomies even if I'm a candidate for breast conservation?

Are there any clinical trials that I should consider? If so, can you recommend trials at your institution or elsewhere?

How soon will the surgery or treatment begin?

Do I qualify for gene expression testing, such as Oncotype DX?

What is the expected recovery time from surgery, and what are the risks?

Will I need to stay in the hospital?

If I prefer to stay in the hospital, is that an option?

What are the side effects of recommended treatments such as radiation or medication?

How much time off from work will I need for the surgery or other treatments?

How high are the chances that I can be fully cured?

What should I be doing until I have the surgery or recommended treatments?

What are the chances for high quality of life?

Great resource: https://www.cancer.org/cancer
/breast-cancer/understanding-a-breast-cancer-diagnosis
/questions-to-ask-your-doctor-about-breast-cancer.html.

Many places will provide a folder or binder for you
to keep track of all your reports and paperwork. If they
don't, you might want to create your own. Now with EMR
(electronic medical records), you should have access to all
your information, but it's helpful to keep everything in one
place as you see different providers during your journey.

CHAPTER 4

You Have a Genetic Mutation

Kelly Wilson had a bad feeling about the biopsy, even before she heard the results. She was only forty-two years old, but ever since the day she learned that she had the BRCA1 mutation, she'd feared the worst, having watched her mother go through surgery and chemotherapy for breast cancer when Kelly was a teenager. Even though Kelly was vigilant about doing her imaging to search for a possible cancer, she was not doing all she could to lead a healthy life; she smoked and didn't exercise regularly.

In 2019, Rachel found an abnormal result on Kelly's MRI. A biopsy revealed an "atypical finding" called atypical ductal hyperplasia (ADH). Something wasn't right. Christy would have to do surgery to find out if it was cancer. This concerning finding opened the door to a completely new question: Had the time come for Kelly to do preventive mastectomies? Would lifestyle changes such as quitting smoking and exercising more regularly reduce her risk, or at least make surgery easier?

We discussed the pros and cons with her at length. Mastectomies would not guarantee that she would never get any cancer of any kind, but they would reduce her odds of getting breast cancer so much that she would never have to worry about it again.

Still, she agonized for months. The argument for preventive mastectomies made sense on paper. But these were *her breasts* we were talking about! Was she willing to remove a body part that was important to her because statistics showed the odds were against her? What did a 30 to 40 percent risk mean, anyway? Maybe she was in the 60 to 70 percent group. Was she willing to gamble her life on that?

Kelly had concerns about what the impact of the surgery might be. She had heard that the expanders doctors used to prepare the chest for implants looked strange, like bricks underneath the skin, and that stressed her. On some level, Kelly knew she wanted to do preventive mastectomies, but she felt so anxious, she kept putting it off. Sometimes facts and statistics have less influence than the things that bother us. In the meantime, she quit smoking and joined a gym, since she could control those aspects of her life.

She finally worked up the nerve to schedule surgery for March 2020. But it had to be canceled at the last moment due to the outbreak of COVID-19, when the onset of the pandemic meant the cancellation of all elective cases.

With all the uncertainties of the pandemic and lockdown on top of waiting for surgery, Kelly took up smoking again. When we finally started doing elective surgeries again in June 2020, we were hesitant to do hers. Ideally, we would've waited three months after she stopped smoking for the effects of nicotine and other toxins in cigarettes to subside. But since she hadn't been smoking very long, the decision was to proceed with surgery as soon as the plastic surgeon felt it was safe. We didn't know what was going to happen with the pandemic, and Kelly was anxious to get the surgery done.

Even those couple of months of smoking during lockdown were enough to cause complications. Smoking causes blood vessels to narrow, which decreases circulation, causing injuries to heal more slowly. This is especially dangerous for people undergoing surgery. During the mastectomies, Kelly's skin showed ischemia, which meant the blood flow to the skin was less than normal. She was able to have expanders (the first step in the reconstructive process for women getting implants—more about that later) placed, but as a result of the ischemia, she had to stay a little longer in the hospital for hyperbaric oxygen therapy. Ultimately, she healed and was able to have the expanders replaced with permanent implants several months later.

With her new implants, Kelly has put all that stress and anxiety behind her. She's getting used to her new breasts, which look great but don't feel natural to her. This was not a surprise since she knew that implants would not feel like her breasts and that there would be numbness. In retrospect, she's happy she decided not to gamble with her life, and that she's one of the lucky ones who had the opportunity to take control and potentially change the course of her life. Maybe she would've been one of the lucky ones and never gotten breast cancer if she hadn't undergone prophylactic mastectomies, but who knows? And now, despite her BRCA1 mutation, she no longer has the anxiety of imaging every six months or the concern about getting breast cancer.

WHO SHOULD GET TESTED AND WHEN?

The genetic mutations most commonly associated with breast cancer are BRCA1 and BRCA2. If either of your parents has one of these variants, you have a 50 percent chance of inheriting it, regardless of your sex or the sex of the parent who carries the gene—which means you can get the gene from your father just as easily as your mother. As a result, half the people with BRCA mutations are male. A BRCA mutation also elevates the risk of other cancers in men, like prostate and colon cancer as well as breast cancer, but the overall risk remains very low—only about 1 percent of breast cancers occur in cisgender men (men born as men).

If you're a woman and have one of the BRCA mutations, your lifetime risk of breast cancer is 50 to 80 percent. You're more likely to get cancer than not. We don't say this to frighten or depress you but instead to empower you. Knowing the statistics can help you make plans that support your health. But testing is far from universal, and many people don't have an accurate accounting of their family's medical history. Some women were adopted or have an adopted parent, and a pattern of cancer can be harder to see in families that are small or primarily male. Previous generations may have been too tactful to say that their great-aunt died of ovarian cancer, that their uncle was suffering from breast cancer, or that the pancreatic disease that killed their grandmother so suddenly was cancer. Even in our more candid times, it's easy to miss a pattern of so many different types of cancer in our extended families. Many learn about cancers their relatives had after being diagnosed with breast cancer, or having a scare. Older generations don't always share cancer diagnoses with family members.

You may already know of a pattern in your own family. If you don't, it's worth doing some research. Knowing can make all the difference. It allows you to take action against a disease that may have attacked your family for generations.[1] You're in a better position than any of them were. We've never had better ways to combat breast cancer than we have today.

It's not necessary for everyone to get genetic testing. The Mayo Clinic encourages testing only for those who have had a breast cancer diagnosis, an ovarian cancer diagnosis, or two or more cancers of any kind themselves. If you have a relative with a BRCA1 or BRCA2 mutation, or if two or more relatives have had BRCA-associated cancers (such as breast cancer, pancreatic cancer, or prostate cancer), it's also a good idea to be tested.[2] However, many providers feel that all members of high-risk populations, like women with a strong family history of breast cancer or a history of atypia or who have had radiation for Hodgkin's lymphoma, should be tested. Still others feel that every woman should be given the opportunity to test for genetic mutations that increase their risk of breast cancer so they can be proactive and consider prophylactic mastectomies should they have a mutation. Dr. Mary-Claire King proposes that screening should be offered to all women around the age of thirty: "To identify a woman as a carrier only after she develops cancer is a failure of cancer prevention."[3] With the readily available genetic tests, any women or man who wants to be tested should be. You'll find more about how to get tested later in this chapter.

We now know that there are many mutations that increase the risk for breast cancer. In addition to BRCA1 and BRCA2, other genetic mutations that increase risk include ATM, TP53, CHEK2, PTEN, CDH1, STK11, and PALB2, among many others. The recommendations regarding surveillance (how to screen in high-risk people) and preventive surgery for each of these mutations depends on when family members were diagnosed with breast cancer and are more individualized than for patients with a BRCA mutation. Unlike BRCA, which has a definitive known risk, other mutations are still being studied to more exactly determine what the chance is that a woman with that mutation will develop breast cancer. As is often the case, recommendations are very personal and individualized.

If you do have a BRCA or other mutation that increases your risk, we also recommend these tests (as was discussed in chapter 2):

- **Magnetic resonance imaging (MRI):** Every year starting at the age of twenty-five.
- **Mammograms:** Every year, at six-month intervals to the MRI, starting at the age of thirty.

- **Ultrasounds:** Many women, and in particular young women, have dense breast tissue that makes mammograms alone more difficult to interpret. Often 3D ultrasounds are the best option (though they don't preclude the need for mammograms). Regardless of genetic status, women with dense breast tissue benefit from annual screening ultrasounds to find the smallest, most curable breast cancers.
- **Biopsies:** As needed. It's not uncommon for imaging findings to require confirmation with ultrasounds. If there's still any question, the tissue will be tested with a biopsy to determine if cancer is present. A biopsy is a sign that your radiologist is doing a thorough evaluation, not that you have cancer. In fact, in 75 to 80 percent of breast biopsies, the result is benign (not cancer). Biopsies are performed to find early, curable breast cancer.

With so much additional scanning, women often ask us if they should be concerned about the exposure to radiation. It's a good question, but nothing to worry about. As the name implies, MRI uses a magnetic field, along with radio waves, to take images. An ultrasound uses sound waves, like sonar and radar. Neither of these tests use ionizing radiation. In fact, the same type of ultrasound is used for breast cancer screening as is used to image babies in utero when a woman is pregnant.

Like X-rays, CT scans, and PET scans, mammograms do use radiation, but the amount is very small—just 0.4 millisieverts (mSv), about the same exposure you'd get during a one-way flight from Chicago to London.[4] In our everyday lives, we're typically exposed to about 3.0 mSv of background radiation a year.[5] Although we're not aware of it, radiation is naturally present in the minerals in our soil and water. About 5 percent of our daily exposure comes from cosmic radiation emanating from the sun and stars, depending on where you live. A year at higher elevations, like in Denver, Colorado, exposures you to 0.8 mSv of cosmic radiation. At sea level, the annual level of cosmic radiation is just 0.3 mSv.[6]

Considering how important regular mammograms are to cancer surveillance, this small amount of radiation is worth it. It's far below the threshold of what our bodies absorb on an ordinary basis. Notably, many studies have shown that there may not be any adverse effect from low-dose radiation, such as the background radiation discussed above, or the radiation of a mammogram. Indeed, these studies strongly support a threshold concept: until a threshold of exposure to radiation is reached, there's no harmful effect from it. Since we aren't certain what that threshold is, we always try to minimize exposure to radiation, but it's certainly lower than background radiation or the radiation from mammography.

WHAT ARE BRCA1 AND BRCA2?

The two most prominent genetic mutations that increase the risk of breast, ovarian, colon, and prostate cancer are known as breast cancer (BRCA) genes 1 and 2. Normally, both genes prevent cancer by repairing breaks in our DNA that make us more likely to get cancer, preventing abnormal cell growth and stabilizing the DNA. In a healthy state, they actively suppress tumors. But if a mutation occurs, these genes don't function properly.

BRCA genes are called tumor suppressor genes, meaning they code for a protein that prevents cells from becoming cancer. Cells are always dividing, and sometimes the division is imperfect, resulting in a faulty cell—a cancer cell. These tumor suppressor proteins clean out abnormal cancer cells, helping prevent breast cancer. However, when these genes are abnormal themselves, the proteins they make are faulty, and they don't stop abnormal cells from growing out of control. We each have two copies of these genes—one from our mother and one from our father. As mentioned earlier, this means we can get a BRCA mutation from either parent. If we inherit an abnormal copy of this gene from one of our parents, the second copy works well—until we get older and a mutation occurs in the second gene. Then there's no protein to prevent cancer cells from dividing, and as a result, breast cancer or other cancers occur.

It's important to note that up to 80 percent of women with the BRCA1 gene get breast cancer—but that means 20 percent do not. There are studies underway to try to understand what protects these BRCA-positive women from getting breast cancer; perhaps we can use that information to prevent breast cancer in other women with the mutation as well. And the different mutations are associated with different cancers. For example, men with the BRCA1 gene have a lower risk of breast cancer than those with the BRCA2 gene, but they have a higher risk of prostate cancer.

Most cases of breast cancer are not caused by BRCA mutations, and as we just mentioned, not everyone with a mutation will develop cancer.[7] However, if your BRCA genes aren't working to repair your DNA, you're significantly more vulnerable, and so are your children, who inherit the gene from you. Without either mutation, you'd have a 12 percent chance of developing breast cancer in the course of your life. With a mutation, your risk of getting breast cancer quintuples.[8]

Cancer caused by BRCA1 mutations is more often found in younger women than cancer caused by BRCA2. It can appear early—even before the recommended screening ages—and it's more challenging to treat. When this mutation causes cancer, it's often triple-negative breast cancer (see page 45), which may not respond to drugs and hormonal treatments as well as other breast cancers, for which there is targeted therapy. Cancers from BRCA2 mutations tend to present a little later, are more likely to be hormone positive, and are generally more responsive to treatment.[9]

There are clearly racial, ethnic, and geographical variations of these genes. In 2019, the largest study ever done using next-generation rapid gene sequencing (NGS) for 35,409 women around the world found 3,000 BRCA1 variants and 3,400 BRCA2 variants.[10] In the United States alone, distinctive BRCA1 variants have been found in African American women; for women of Ashkenazi Jewish descent, there are a number of different mutations of the BRCA1 and two mutations for the BRCA2 genes.[11] In some communities, the gene is much more frequent, such as the Ashkenazi Jewish community, where the gene is found ten times more frequently than in the general population.

The human genome has 6.4 billion base pairs—and we only confirmed that in 2003. We still have a lot to learn about our genes! For all the new research about BRCA, less than half (48.5 percent) of the genes associated with breast cancer in that 2019 study were BRCA genes or variants.[12] That's why knowing your family history can really help fill in the gaps. In addition, discussions with a genetic counselor can help clarify this complex, ever-changing field. The genetic counselor can also help discuss your risk even if your test results don't demonstrate a genetic mutation but there's a strong family history. This is exactly what happened with Christy, her friend Laurie, and many of our patients. The family or personal history of breast cancer suggests a potential genetic link, but the genetic testing comes back negative. Can we always trust a negative result, or should we assume there may be additional mutations discovered in the future? The answer is undoubtedly yes, since there's no doubt that, with time, more genes associated with an increased risk of many cancers, including breast cancer, will be identified.

GETTING A GENETIC TEST

A simple test can let you know where you stand. Almost all insurance carriers cover the cost of genetic testing for women with a significant family history of cancer or a BRCA mutation, especially when it's recommended by your regular physician, surgeon, oncologist, or genetic counselor. Even if insurance doesn't cover the test, you can have it done at a much more reasonable cost today than in the past. Previously, the cost of genetic testing was often $3,000 or more. Today there are numerous, highly reputable tests that cost approximately $200 to $300. There are also an increasing number of commercially available direct-to-consumer companies that test for genes associated with increased risk of breast cancer. In fact, the field has become much more sophisticated, and many test for other risks as well, including cardiac risk and risk of drug allergies.

Recently, Wendy Dixon, a close friend of Christy's, got an unusual call from her older brother, Jack. He had just gotten his results back from an online genetic service and was startled to learn that he had a BRCA2 mutation. Knowing that the mutation tends to run in families, he called Wendy right away.

For as long as Christy has known her, Wendy has hated seeing doctors. One year, she suffered through a bout of strep throat for days before getting antibiotics. No one was sure if she was tougher than the rest of us or just more afraid of doctors.

This time, because she knew Christy well, she felt more comfortable meeting with her and a genetic counselor. Wendy's parents came along to help her flesh out their family history and to be tested themselves. We wanted to test Wendy and one of her parents for the specific BRCA2 mutation that was found in her brother.

We learned that Wendy's father's father had had breast cancer. There were no women with cancer on that side of the family and no sign of cancer on her mother's side of the family. The genetic counselor tested both Wendy and her father. When the results came back, both Wendy and her father had BRCA2 mutations. Wendy now does regular screenings with mammograms and MRIs and is getting over her fear of doctors.

It's important to note that while the results helped alert Wendy, Jack, and their father to a risk they'd never suspected, consumer testing isn't the same as a screening with imaging, clinical examination, or consultation with a genetic counselor. With something this pivotal to your health, we strongly recommend seeing a trained professional for further guidance. This includes a genetic counselor, an oncologist, or a high-risk surveillance program, so that if the tests do demonstrate a genetic mutation associated with an increased risk of breast cancer, someone is there to help guide you with regard to next steps and surveillance strategies. Even when online genetic tests are accurate, they don't let you know what to do with the information you receive.

When the test is evaluated by a physician or a genetic counselor, you can learn whether you're at increased risk. Because genetic counselors are trained to take extensive family histories and make nuanced connections, they're uniquely qualified to identify mutations that might be missed by consumer lab tests. This is important, because genetic tests don't test for all genetic mutations associated with an increased risk for cancer; rather, the genetic counselor requests a certain battery of tests for specific genes. Genetic testing won't tell you whether you already have the disease (clinical validity). You will, however, be armed with critical information to obtain further invaluable information about prevention, diagnosis, management, or treatment of the disease (clinical usefulness).[13]

You can make an appointment for testing with a referral from your doctor, or reach out to a genetic counselor yourself. The genetic counselor will take an extensive, detailed family history and make subtle but important connections in order to ensure your test includes a search for all genes that may affect your breast cancer risk (at least, all the ones current science knows to look for) and thereby request the best test for you. They'll prepare you for your test and get insurance approval. The test itself usually requires only a single small vial of blood or a saliva sample. The results typically come back in about three weeks. When they come in, you'll meet again with the genetic counselor, who's trained to help you process the information and help you with your reaction to the test results.

If your test is negative, it means that no mutation was detected. The best news you could get is a "true negative": when a family member has cancer with a specific mutation and you don't have that mutation, it means you don't have that particular risk. It's certainly worthy of a big sigh of relief. It's no guarantee that you won't get cancer, of course. None of us have that. But finding out that you eluded a family mutation is cause for celebration.

If you test positive for a genetic mutation, it doesn't mean you have cancer. It means you have an increased risk for getting breast cancer in the future. Having a genetic counselor at your side when you learn this information is enormously helpful. They can explain the implications of the results for you and your family, so you can make informed decisions about what happens next. Your counselor will discuss any doubts, concerns, or fears you may have at the time or if you have questions later. It's always better to ask than to worry. The better informed you are, the better you can cope with whatever reality you face. The genetic counselors can explain your risks and recommend an effective surveillance program or direct you to a high-risk professional or clinic. It's hard to find out you have a gene mutation without a professional who can guide you through what to do next. If you do find out that you have a mutation through a commercial laboratory, you should seek out a high-risk program near you where there's a co-ordinated team to help with the information, surveillance strategies, and information and expertise about prophylactic surgery, should you be interested in pursuing that.

When you have a BRCA mutation, your three best options are:

- **Surveillance,** which can identify cancer at the earliest possible stage. This includes mammography, ultrasound, and MRI. The goal here is to find cancer at its most curable stage. Surveillance was discussed earlier in this chapter and in more detail in chapter 2.
- **Preventive mastectomy,** which is the removal of healthy breasts. The goal with this approach is to prevent you from ever getting breast cancer and to change the narrative of your and your family's futures. This was discussed in this chapter and throughout the book.
- **Chemoprevention,** which means reducing the risk of getting breast cancer by taking medications rather than having surgery. This involves taking a drug such as tamoxifen to block estrogen. This will be discussed later in this chapter and in chapter 5. This approach does decrease your risk of breast cancer, but by far less than prophylactic mastectomy.

We've never had as many realizable screening options for those with breast cancer–related mutations as we have today. Our ability to detect breast cancer early has improved dramatically in the past decade alone. With regular screening, we can identify and test anything that even *might* be cancer. Early detection means your treatment can be less aggressive and your recovery time much shorter. The screening process is far less stressful when you have a good relationship with your doctor, who specializes in caring for high-risk patients, and your radiologist. Like the genetic counselor, they can inform you, allay your fears, and help you put your results in perspective.

INTERVENTION WITH PREVENTIVE (ALSO CALLED PROPHYLACTIC) MASTECTOMIES

Nobody wants to remove healthy breasts. But in our practices, we find that many women with genetic mutations choose to do so when the alternative is gambling on the terrible odds of getting cancer. As this book shows, we believe that for the right women, preventive mastectomies offer the greatest protection and peace of mind.

Women with a positive test result for BRCA1 or BRCA2 or other mutations that increase their risk for breast cancer will also find that doctors don't hesitate to encourage this step. They won't have to argue their case for preventive mastectomies. Physicians experienced in caring for high-risk patients will help guide women through the multiple decisions and process involved.

The decision to remove diseased breast tissue is straightforward; the choice of whether and when to take away beautiful healthy breasts is much more complicated and difficult. To many women, our breasts are so much more than just a body part: they're a living symbol of our womanhood, a private pleasure for ourselves and our partners, a reminder of the children we've nursed (or hope to nurse). They make us feel beautiful, or simply feel like ourselves, and we fear we will lose something more than flesh if they're taken from us. So many conflicting emotions come into play when you're asked to choose between two profoundly terrible options: removing your breasts, or risking the high probability of breast cancer. It's hardly fair, but knowing your risk and having control over the outcome is empowering. If you've had loved ones who suffered with or died from cancer, the decision is often easier. But even then, it's strongly affected by whether you're single or in a relationship, whether you've already had children or hope to have them later, and whether you're more frightened by surveillance or can tolerate your greater risk of cancer. It's a very personal decision, with no right or wrong answer. Every person is different, and every decision is influenced by a woman's experiences and life situation. Not every woman copes with risk in the same way.

We can't tell you whether you—you personally, you specifically—should or should not have preventive mastectomies if you discover you have a genetic mutation that puts you at high risk. But we can hold your hand (figuratively) and walk you through the factors to consider as you make the decision.

For women with a BRCA mutation, the risk for developing breast cancer is between 50 to 80 percent. If you remove both breasts, you reduce your risk of breast cancer to as low as 2 percent, which is lower than the average American woman's risk of 12 percent. When it comes to genetic mutations specifically, women with a BRCA mutation who have been diagnosed with breast cancer have a much higher risk of developing another breast cancer later, either on the same side or in the opposite breast.

Are there any other statistics women should know to help make this huge decision, particularly those with genetic predisposition? For example, does family history interact with BRCA mutations, or is it a binary thing? In other words, should someone positive for BRCA mutations but with very little family history of cancer be thinking about this the same way as someone positive with an extensive family history? Should readers like Emily in the story that follows be thinking about a certain age for preventive mastectomy? What questions should patients discuss with physicians, and what factors tend to sway them most strongly one way or another?

As it turns out, the same mutation has different effects in different women. Medical research increasingly shows that a number of variables, such as the age of family members when they were diagnosed, can modify the risk for women with mutations. Cancer develops from a complex interaction of genes. The balance between the negative impact of the gene and the body's ability to respond to the gene consequence varies with each individual. That's why some women with BRCA mutations get cancer in their twenties, and some with the same exact mutation never get cancer.

For women who test positive for a mutation, it's reasonable to consider surveillance, or intense screening, instead of bilateral preventive mastectomies. The choice of bilateral preventive mastectomies, even in women with genetic mutations, is extremely personal, but for the right women, the decision to undergo preventive mastectomies is no longer radical.

Since statistics can only tell you what happened to other people, not what will happen to you, it all comes down to hope. You choose surveillance because you hope to find cancer early, if it occurs. You choose preventive mastectomies because you hope to escape breast cancer altogether.

When Christy first saw Emily Jensen, Emily was thirty-two years old and had tested positive for a BRCA2 mutation. It was no surprise. Both her mother and her grandfather had died of breast cancer when they were in their sixties. We spent a long time discussing the pros and cons of surveillance vs. preventive mastectomies. She liked the idea of reducing her odds of getting breast cancer with mastectomies, but she didn't want to do it right away.

"I love my breasts!" she said. "I want to enjoy them as long as I possibly can. My mother didn't get cancer until she was fifty, so I've got a little time, don't I?"

"As long as you're willing to do the surveillance," I told her, "and assume the risk."

She was. For eight years, she faithfully showed up for scans and tests with little to no anxiety. She didn't mind spending an hour at the hospital for imaging a few times a year. She never needed any biopsies for suspicious lumps and didn't stress out while she waited for the results. When she turned forty, she scheduled preventive mastectomies, giving her mother's age of diagnosis a ten-year margin just in case.

Emily's new breasts are not exactly like her original breasts, but she has the same nipples and the implants gave her a slightly larger size, which she enjoys. (We will talk in more detail about the options for surgery, including nipple-sparing techniques, in chapter 8.) Most of all, being informed and objectively evaluating the odds gave her confidence. Not only did she avoid breast cancer, she was also able to assert some agency and control over a situation that had carried fear and grief for her and her family.

Confronting a high risk of breast cancer is difficult. There is no easy out. But genetic testing can serve as an early-warning system, allowing you to choose between more and better options than are available after diagnosis. It gives you control.

Maria Thompson knew her family had a strong history of ovarian cancer on her father's side. She was relieved to learn that they had no history of breast cancer at all, although several relatives had tested positive for a BRCA2 mutation. Maria tested positive for the same mutation.

To be on the safe side, she opted for preventive surgery to have both of her ovaries removed (known as bilateral oophorectomies) by the time she was forty-five. Removing her ovaries reduced her risk of getting breast cancer by around 50 percent. She's considering preventive mastectomies, too, but with no breast cancer in her family, she isn't inclined to do it.

Another option we discussed was for Maria to take preventive hormonal treatments. An estrogen modulator, such as tamoxifen, or an aromatase inhibitor could potentially reduce her risk further. I explained that there tend to be fewer serious side effects with aromatase inhibitors than with tamoxifen, which can cause strokes, blood clots, and endometrial cancer. On the other hand, heart issues, bone loss, and osteoporosis are far more common with aromatase inhibitors.[14] Maria elected not to take any medications since removing her ovaries had already reduced her risk significantly. She's content to continue with surveillance, knowing that she has the option of having preventive surgery at any time if she changes her mind.

Dora Schoenberg was in her thirties when she found out that she had a BRCA1 mutation. She was aware that she may decide eventually to have preventive oophorectomies and mastectomies, but she felt confident in the efficacy of diligent surveillance. Every six months for ten years, she appeared for either a mammogram or an MRI without incident. We've often discussed how fortunate we are to have excellent screening options for breast cancer, although the same isn't true for ovarian cancer. Dora is very grateful to have avoided surgery for so long.

Over the years, she has had to undergo several biopsies due to false positive results from breast MRIs. She isn't eager to go through that again, but that unpleasant experience is still not enough to outweigh removing her breasts.

Now, at the age of forty-two, she's considering removing her ovaries. While MRIs for breast cancer can yield false positive results, ultrasounds and bloodwork for ovarian cancer can often provide false negative results, so the risk of surveillance for ovarian cancer is much greater. Dora is aware of the dangers of waiting. While avoiding regular scans, bloodwork, and biopsies is appealing, she knows that surgery also comes with risks, recovery time, and, in some cases, follow-up surgeries and adjustment periods. She's also aware that there's no guarantee that cancer won't happen while she's undergoing surveillance. It isn't an easy decision from any point of view.

In contrast to Dora, one of our other patients, Ashley Brown, found out that she had a BRCA1 mutation at the age of thirty-four and was anxious to have both preventive mastectomies and oophorectomies. She was fine with doing screening with Rachel, and had just had a normal MRI, but she didn't want to worry about breast or ovarian cancer. She had multiple family members who had had breast and ovarian cancer. When she saw Christy, she was trying to figure out the best timing. Christy suggested doing the mastectomies first. That way, Ashley wouldn't have to worry about taking hormones to avoid menopausal symptoms when her ovaries were removed. She liked that idea, and proceeded with bilateral mastectomies with reconstruction. In the final pathology, an early noninvasive cancer was found in one of her breasts. Several months later, she had her ovaries removed and was able to take hormone replacement therapy, since the cancer found in her breast was not invasive.

You may be facing the same conundrum. Even if you ultimately never get breast cancer, facing the prospect of cancer with honesty, as these women did, requires great courage and strength. In our practice, we've seen thousands of women rise to this challenge, despite their fears and anxieties. Thanks to the remarkable medical advances we can employ today, we've seen so many of our patients live longer, healthier lives than was ever possible before. We feel very honored that they've trusted us with their care.

Common Questions to Discuss with Your Care Team

How is genetic testing done? Will my insurance cover it?

What kind of information will a genetic test provide?

How soon will I get the results?

Will I be told the results by phone or at my next appointment?

Should I meet with a genetic counselor to discuss the results?

What do my results mean for the members of my family?

If I test positive, does that mean my family members are at higher risk, too?

What do I tell family members who aren't interested in being tested?

Does a positive test put me at risk for discrimination or future insurance issues?

If I test positive, what's my risk for developing breast cancer?

If I test negative, does that mean I'm not at an increased risk for developing breast cancer?

How can I decrease my risk of getting breast cancer if I do test positive?

What additional screening do I need to do if I test positive, and where should I have it done?

Who do you recommend I see to discuss risk-reduction surgery?

If genetic testing shows that I have a mutation, am I at increased risk of other cancers?

Does a positive genetic test mean I'm more likely to have a recurrence of breast cancer?

Is it possible for the results of a genetic test to be uncertain?

My genetic test came back with something called a "variant of unknown significance." What does that mean for me?

Will I need to take a genetic test again in the future?

CHAPTER 5

You Have an Increased Risk for Breast Cancer

Preventive mastectomies are now widely accepted for women with a BRCA mutation, since the risk can be clearly verified with a genetic test. But what about the many women with a strong family history of breast cancer with no confirmed mutation? Do we know for sure that their risk of developing breast cancer is any less?

Many of the factors that increase our risk of getting cancer of any kind are still unknown. With significant medical research devoted to the discovery of the causes, influences, and markers that lead to cancer, we're making progress toward better insights and more effective treatments every year.

In this chapter, we will highlight four risks in particular. We already know that family history can be a significant risk factor. Women with particularly dense breasts are also at greater risk. If your doctor takes a series of biopsies with findings called atypia, or atypical cells, you should be aware that this can increase your risk of breast cancer, too. More rarely, if you've been treated with radiation for Hodgkin's lymphoma, your risk of breast cancer may have tripled as a result of that treatment, which includes radiation to the area of the breasts.

We will also discuss various risk-assessment tools used to help determine a woman's risk for developing breast cancer in the next five years, as well as her lifetime risk. The results help clinicians determine future screening and best methods for risk reduction for each individual patient.

The essential question in a book about mastectomies and risk-based screening is whether these increased risks—perhaps less definitive than a lab result in black and white—warrant consideration of removing your breasts. How can you possibly know unless you truly understand the nature of the risk you're facing? Many of these issues are not openly discussed, even when you ask frank questions of your own doctors and oncologists. Our desire to help you evaluate your situation and make an informed choice is what this book is about.

A strong family history was warning enough for Christy to consider and ultimately go forward with preventive mastectomies. Even though her mother's genetic tests showed that she didn't have one of the BRCA mutations, Christy was concerned that the cause of her mother's cancer could have been genetic, especially since her mother's second cancer was so aggressive, and her mother's aunt had died from breast cancer at an early age. She simply didn't want to take the chance.

In our experience, women who work in medicine and are either diagnosed with breast cancer or at an increased risk for it—with or without genetic mutations—are often very proactive about having preventive mastectomies. Maybe it's because we see firsthand the impact that breast cancer has on our patients, our friends, our families, and sometimes ourselves. Maybe it's the often painful choices, or the disappointment when important plans are disrupted by the ugly face of cancer, or maybe it's the time crunch if cancer is diagnosed, the need to make decisions quicker than you would with the luxury of time. Perhaps we want control. Maybe it's all of this. That's exactly what happened with Christy. After watching her best friend Laurie go through chemotherapy twice and experience all the side effects, lose the job that she loved when she was in the middle of treatments after her second diagnosis, and struggle to find another job after having her mastectomies, Christy was going to be sure she had complete control and avoided the risk of getting cancer. Because the surgery was preventive and elective, Christy was free to have mastectomies at a time that was right for her work and family. As a result, she felt empowered.

If you're at risk for getting breast cancer, there are ways to minimize that risk, to some degree. General lifestyle changes, such as diet and exercise, can certainly improve your health and boost your immune system, and medications such as tamoxifen can also reduce your risk. But the most definitive way to significantly reduce your risk of breast cancer is to remove your breasts altogether with preventive mastectomies. It's neither an easy decision nor an easy procedure or recovery, but neither of us have heard of women who have regretted it. Many love their new breasts, like Christy and Rachel do. Some may not love their new breasts—or lack of them, for those who elect against reconstruction—but in our experience, all are thankful to no longer have to worry about getting breast cancer.

1. YOUR FAMILY HISTORY

The best-known genes associated with an increased risk of breast cancer are BRCA1 and BRCA2. We tend to think of them as two simple mutations, but the reality is far more complicated than that. In fact, there are more than twenty thousand unique variations of BRCA1 and BRCA2 genes. So far, the National Cancer Program of the NIH has determined that at least 3,700 of them cause disease. There are over seventy other genes besides BRCA that have been identified as having an association with an increased risk of breast cancer. There are undoubtedly many more that haven't yet been identified. As studies progress and with the availability of large data sets worldwide, the number will continue to increase.[1] It's certainly possible that a strong prevalence of cancer within a family can occur from environmental toxins; in these cases, multiple families from the same area with a high prevalence of cancer can often be identified. It's far more likely that a family with a history of cancer may have a genetic proclivity that we simply haven't yet discovered.

A large number of women who have a strong family history of breast cancer concerning a genetic mutation continue to test negative; they're known as BRCAX.[2] The women in this group are presumed to have a genetic predisposition for breast cancer, but the specific genetic mutation hasn't been identified (the "X" in BRCAX refers to the unknown mutation). But in just the past five years, we've made enormous progress in identifying mutations associated with breast cancer. If you tested negative and the tests were done more than five years ago, it's worth getting retested. Of course, no test exists that can find all the mutations that increase a woman's chance of breast cancer.[3] We still don't even know what they all are. What we do know is that a family history of breast cancer significantly increases your risk. The data is very clear: If your mother, sister, or daughter (first-degree relatives) was diagnosed with breast cancer, your risk doubles. Two first-degree relatives with breast cancer increases your risk three times.[4]

One way to protect yourself if any of your relatives have been diagnosed with breast cancer before the age of fifty is to start getting mammograms ten years before the age of their diagnosis or at age of forty, whichever comes first. If your calculated risk of breast cancer is a lifetime risk of 20 percent or greater, add annual MRI screenings, generally separated from the time of your mammogram by six months so that you're seen twice a year.

Another of Christy's patients, Maria Perez, had an abnormal finding on her imaging, which required a breast biopsy. Although her results were not worrisome, Maria was extremely stressed. Now in her thirties, she had watched her sister suffer through chemotherapy and mastectomies at an early age and had found the experience traumatic. The possibility that she may have cancer was very frightening, and waiting for the biopsy results was agonizing for her.

Every six months, Maria alternated MRIs with mammograms, according to the standard protocol, but in her case, the MRIs often turned up suspicious findings that led to more biopsies. Each one was nerve-racking for her and brought back the emotions she had felt during her sister's cancer.

Years later, when an MRI showed findings in both breasts that needed further testing and evaluation, Maria decided it was time to have preventive mastectomies. The stress of anticipating the biopsies, the discomfort of the procedures, and her anxiety while waiting for the results was too difficult. She was tired of living in fear of going through her sister's experience, and she didn't want to worry anymore.

She had bilateral nipple-sparing mastectomies, and our plastic surgeon reconstructed her breasts with implants. Maria was very happy with the results, and was hugely relieved that she no longer had to endure the stress that mammograms and MRIs caused for her.

As a result of her experience, she decided to become a nurse to give back. Five years after surgery, she often takes care of Christy's patients when they're admitted after surgery. When Christy and Maria run into each other at the hospital, Maria is still full of emotion, but now she sheds tears of joy and relief. She is indeed giving back and helping our patients in so many ways.

2. DENSE BREASTS

Aside from family history, dense breast tissue is another common cause of increased breast cancer risk.[5] Since breasts are made up of breast tissue and fat, it's the percentage of breast tissue that determines breast density. How your breasts look or feel won't tell you whether they're dense. We aren't talking about firmness or sagginess. The density of tissue can only be determined on a mammogram, which uses ionizing radiation.

The American College of Radiology classifies 50 percent or more breast tissue as dense (either C or D density).[6] Fortunately, breast density decreases with age, but it's often an issue throughout a woman's life. Seventy percent of women in their forties have dense breast tissue, and 30 percent still do in their seventies.[7]

Dense breast tissue is the perfect storm, creating a higher risk of breast cancer, but a reduced ability to see the cancer with a mammogram. Mammograms detect 85 percent of breast cancer,[8] but in women with dense breast tissue, approximately 50 percent of cancers are not visible on a mammogram.[9] On a mammogram, breast tissue is white and breast cancers are white. There isn't enough contrast to differentiate between them. In women with dense breast tissue, the cancers that are hidden are mostly small, invasive, node-negative cancer—the most potentially lethal cancers. Because they're so hard to detect with mammography alone, breast cancers in women with dense breast tissue are often diagnosed later, after they have spread to the lymph nodes. To make matters worse, women with dense breast tissue are more likely to have interval cancers, those diagnosed within a year of a normal mammogram and felt by the woman or her healthcare provider, not discovered during their next mammogram. Interval cancers have a worse prognosis that those detected by a mammogram.

As many as 40 percent of women in the US have dense breasts.[10] Women with extremely dense breasts are at a four to six times greater risk of developing breast cancer.[11] This is why women who do have dense breast tissue need additional essential screening to improve the odds of detecting cancer at its earliest, most curable stage. Having dense breast tissue doesn't mean that prophylactic mastectomy is indicated. In fact, dense breasts alone are not enough of a risk factor for someone to undergo prophylactic mastectomy. However, additional screening with annual ultrasound or even MRI is essential. Recent studies have shown that in women with extremely dense breasts, MRI is the imaging modality that finds the most breast cancers.[12]

Rachel is often asked if there's a way younger women can determine their breast density without the ionizing radiation of a mammogram. Recently, the FDA cleared SoftVue ultrasound tomography, an exciting new technology that uses ultrasound to find additional cancers in women with dense breast tissue. It can also determine a woman's breast density without exposing patients to ionizing radiation. Hopefully, we will soon be able to have this technology in the clinic; at the time of this writing, however, breast density can only be determined by a mammogram.

Dense breast tissue is also a political issue. Every mammogram report must describe breast density; this is mandated by law. Thirty-eight states and the District of Columbia now have laws that require that women be informed by their radiologist about their breast density. Rachel is proud that the Brem Foundation to Defeat Breast Cancer was instrumental in the writing and passage of the Breast Density Screening and Notification Amendment Act of 2018 in the District of Columbia, which mandates insurance coverage of the essential tests to find additional cancers in women with dense breast tissue. However, every state with a law like this uses different language: some only require telling a woman that she has dense breast tissue, some require informing women that additional testing can find cancers hidden in the dense breast tissue, and some require insurance coverage of these essential (not additional) tests. The FDA has proposed federally standardized language about dense breast tissue. Although this is an excellent effort, it does not, in our opinion, go far enough to inform women with dense breast tissue of the additional tests they need, which include annual bilateral ultrasounds in addition to their mammogram. Some women with dense breasts may undergo annual MRI instead of ultrasound, since MRI finds the most cancers. However, not all insurance companies will cover annual MRI, and there's the possibility of the accumulation of gadolinium, a contrast agent often used with MRI, in the brain (see page 31). However, if a woman has an annual MRI to screen for breast cancer, she may not also need ultrasound. So women with dense breasts should at least have an annual screening ultrasound; others may need breast MRIs, particularly if they have a family history of breast cancer or other risk factors.

The National Cancer Institute has designated multiple cancer centers in the US as comprehensive cancer centers. These centers make up the National Comprehensive Cancer Network (NCCN), which establishes guidelines for patients undergoing treatment for breast cancer and for those at risk for developing it. It also includes guidelines for any patients with a Gail model five-year risk greater than 1.7 percent or a lifetime risk greater than 20 percent, as well as patients with a family history of breast cancer. (The Gail model, along with other risk calculators, are described later in this chapter.) The guidelines are not only for screening but also for discussions about risk reduction, including chemoprevention with tamoxifen, aromatase inhibitors, or

Evista (raloxifene, a selective estrogen receptor modulator [SERM] like tamoxifen that is more commonly used for treating patients with osteopenia or osteoporosis), or the option of prophylactic surgery. It also includes lifestyle modifications, such as assessing the number of years on hormone replacement therapy, exercise, weight control, and alcohol consumption. If you would like to know more about breast density, please visit the Brem Foundation website, bremfoundation.org, or see the NCCN's guidelines at www .nccn.org/guidelines/patients.

Although dense breast tissue is an important and frequent risk factor for developing breast cancer, it isn't in and of itself a reason to undergo preventive mastectomies. Rather, it's something every woman should know about herself in order to be fully prepared and should insist on the additional testing that's needed to optimally screen for early, curable breast cancer. In women with dense breast tissue, mammography isn't enough. Additional essential screening with ultrasound or, in certain cases, MRI is needed to find breast cancers that hide in dense tissue. This additional screening ensures that we can find the earliest, most curable breast cancer in women with dense breast tissue.

3. BIOPSIES WITH ATYPICAL FINDINGS

When Erica Stevens was forty, scans showed unusual findings in her right breast. The biopsy showed that she had some abnormal cells in the duct that carries milk from the lobules (milk sacs) to the nipples. The cells differed from normal cells but were not abnormal enough to be cancer; they were "atypical," which means not typical or not completely normal. Because the condition occurs in the ducts of the breast, it's called atypical ductal hyperplasia (ADH), which literally means "an unusual proliferation of cells in the ducts." When these atypical cells are seen in the lobules, it's called atypical lobular hyperplasia (ALH).

When atypical cells are found on a needle biopsy, we recommend that the woman undergo surgical excision to be certain that the adjacent cells are not cancer, which they are in anywhere from 5 to 25 percent of cases.[13] There is agreement that all women with ADH have surgical excision. The situation with ALH isn't as straightforward, and while some institutions do recommend surgical excision of ALH, some do not. However, the data is compelling that there's a substantially increased risk of finding cancer at surgical excision with ALH, and therefore, we recommend that all our patients have surgical excision when a needle biopsy determines they have ALH. Having atypical cells, whether ductal or lobular, also substantially increases a woman's lifetime risk of developing breast cancer. Therefore, not only does the tissue in the breast need to be further examined for cancer when ADH or ALH is found to exclude the possibility of adjacent cancer, there's also a substantially increased lifetime risk of developing cancer.

With Erica, we surgically removed the area that showed the atypical cells on biopsy, and the results showed no evidence of cancer. We discussed the option of Erica taking tamoxifen to reduce her elevated breast cancer risk, but she didn't like taking medications and preferred observation. Six months later, her MRI showed an area of enhancement in the left breast, indicating an abnormality that required biopsy to determine whether cancer was present. A subsequent MRI-guided biopsy showed another kind of atypical cells called lobular carcinoma in situ (LCIS). While LCIS has the word "carcinoma" in it, it's not a cancer, but it does require surgical excision to exclude cancer—and it further increased Erica's risk of breast cancer. Erica was adopted, so she had no idea whether her birth family had a history of breast cancer. However, we were concerned that so many unusual findings in such a such short period of time suggested an increased risk of her developing cancer. These "atypical proliferations" that had now been found in her breast twice in less than a year suggested there could be other areas in the breast with similar findings.

Because she didn't have a diagnosis of breast cancer, she took her time to decide what to do. Ultimately, she chose to have bilateral mastectomies with implant reconstruction. Her breasts were too large for nipple-sparing mastectomies, but she loves the smaller size of her breasts and has three-dimensional tattoos that look like nipples with areolas (we talk more about this in chapter 9).

As mentioned, findings such as ADH, ALH, and LCIS can significantly increase a woman's risk of developing breast cancer. Like ADH and ALH, LCIS is a high-risk marker. Surgical excision is recommended to be sure that the adjacent cells are more likely to be cancer. Finding cancer at surgical excision of these high-risk lesions occurs in 5 to 25 percent of women.[14] The risk of developing breast cancer after a diagnosis of LCIS is approximately 2 percent per year.[15] This can translate to an estimated lifetime risk of breast cancer as high as 30 to 40 percent, compared to 12 percent for the general population. The lifetime risk for ADH can be as high as 30 percent.[16]

Women with ADH, ALH, and LCIS are often referred to oncologists to discuss risk reduction strategies, which, as we discussed previously, may include trying to prevent breast cancer with medications such tamoxifen for chemoprevention as it has been shown to reduce the risk for developing breast cancer by as much as 50 percent. The questions to discuss with your oncologists include how much benefit these drugs will give you, what the side effects from the medications are when compared to the reduction in risk, and which drugs are available to you for risk reduction. Every woman's consideration is different. Some will embrace the risks of chemoprevention for the risk reduction, and some will think the risk is tolerable enough to avoid these drugs. Once again, this is a very personal decision, but one you should make fully informed.

4. HODGKIN'S LYMPHOMA

Dory Young was treated for Hodgkin's lymphoma when she was nineteen. Chemotherapy and radiation made it necessary for her to take a year off from college. Afterward, she went on to get her law degree. Twice a year from the time she was thirty, she came back to us for surveillance, with physical exams and mammograms alternating with MRIs.

When she was thirty-seven, her MRI showed a small mass in her right breast. An ultrasound and guided-core needle biopsy showed a very challenging cancer, triple-negative invasive ductal carcinoma. Sadly, 50 percent of patients treated for Hodgkin's lymphoma between the ages of ten and thirty will go on to develop breast cancers, which are often triple-negative, the more aggressive type of breast cancer, generally requiring chemotherapy.[17]

We recommended a nipple-sparing mastectomy on the right, but Dory didn't want to risk having cancer again, so she decided to have mastectomies on both sides. We did the reconstruction using her own abdominal fat, giving her a tummy tuck at the same time (a procedure described in chapter 9).

Because her tumor was triple-negative, chemotherapy was recommended. For women in their forties, having to go through chemotherapy a second time after being treated in their late teens can be devastating.

Dory took it remarkably well. Although she was disappointed to have to go through chemotherapy again, she told herself that she could get through this time, just like she had when she was younger. She took a couple of days off from work after each treatment, but continued working during those four months. This helped to make the time go by more quickly for her, and unlike the last time she had chemotherapy, she was able to keep her hair by using cold caps (described in chapter 3).

The recommendation for women who underwent radiation for Hodgkin's lymphoma between the ages of ten and thirty is to start surveillance, including annual mammograms alternating with MRIs every six months, ten years after their treatment for Hodgkin's. If a woman had Hodgkin's lymphoma later in life, her risk of breast cancer isn't as high. To complicate matters further, there's a lifetime limit on the amount of radiation that any tissue can receive. That's why women who develop breast cancer following radiation for Hodgkin's cannot undergo lumpectomy; since the area of the breast receives some of the radiation during treatment for Hodgkin's, the radiation required following lumpectomy cannot be administered without going over that lifetime limit. Since the risk of breast cancer is nearly as high in these woman as it is in women with genetic mutations, considering preventive mastectomies is reasonable.

HOW MUCH RISK DO YOU FACE?

If you do have one of these four factors that significantly increase your risk of getting breast cancer, the question is, how does it affect your own personal level of risk?

Fortunately, there are several tools that can give you and your doctor insights about this. The Gail model, also known as the Breast Cancer Risk Assessment Tool, was designed by scientists at the National Cancer Institute to assess a woman's risk of developing an invasive breast cancer in the next five years and across her lifetime.[18] It considers your reproductive history, any biopsies you may have had as well as any unusual findings in those biopsies, and any history of breast cancer in your first-degree relatives. (Because it only includes first-degree relatives on your mother's side, it underestimates the risk of cancers from your father's side.)

Women with a known genetic mutation or a history of abnormal cell growth, or who have had radiation for Hodgkin's lymphoma are excluded because their risk is already greater than the 20 percent, so surveillance with annual MRI is always recommended.

When the Gail model determined that our patient Eleanor Stevens had a lifetime risk of developing breast cancer of over 30 percent, she wanted to rethink her options. She had already undergone multiple biopsies and several surgeries for atypical hyperplasia, or unusual cell growth. Eleanor was a scientist, and she felt that a 30 percent risk was greater than what she and her significant other at the time (now her husband) were willing to take. She decided to be proactive and elected to have bilateral preventive mastectomies.

It was 2007, just as the practice of nipple-sparing mastectomies was becoming available. Christy was very interested in offering the option to patients, and Eleanor was willing to be the first! Along with an outstanding plastic surgeon, Christy performed the first nipple-sparing mastectomies with implant reconstructions. Eleanor was very pleased with the results. Since that time, we've performed thousands of nipple-sparing mastectomies, and we're still grateful that Eleanor was willing to be the first. Four years later in 2011, Christy reaped the benefit of having developed an experienced team when she had her own nipple-sparing mastectomies.

The Gail model is one of three assessments we rely on today; the others are the Contraceptive and Reproductive Experiences

(CARE) model and the Tyrer-Cuzick model. All the risk models are questionnaires and are reasonable models for assessing risk. Because they use different metrics, the three models yield different results—sometimes *very* different results—in the same person. It should also be pointed out that none of these models are "right." Rather, they're a method of estimating a woman's risk of breast cancer using population-based knowledge.

The CARE model was developed for risk assessment of African American women. It was added to the Gail model when doctors realized that breast cancer in African American women was being consistently underestimated.[19] There are concerns, however, that the CARE model may still underestimate risk in Black women with previous biopsies or in Hispanic or Latinx women born outside the United States.

The Tyrer-Cuzick model (also known as IBIS) uses both personal and family histories to determine the ten-year and lifetime risks for developing breast cancer. Like the Gail model, it excludes women with a known genetic mutation. Unlike the Gail model, it also includes breast density, family history on the father's side, mothers with bilateral mastectomies, and Ashkenazi Jewish heritage in its assessment.

A study comparing the Gail model to the Tyrer-Cuzick model found that Gail underestimated risk for women with a family history of breast cancer and that Tyrer-Cuzick was more appropriate for risk assessment. (Keep in mind that these risk assessment tools aren't definitive. They're the best tools we have, but they're only aids to help us assess your risks.[20] No tool can say conclusively whether you will get breast cancer.)

The different risk assessment tools are used in various practices to determine a woman's risk for developing breast cancer. Each practice has its favorite test, and one isn't better than the others, but the results can vary. For example, when Christy put her data into the Tyrer-Cuzick software, her lifetime risk was 38 percent, compared to the population's average risk of 10.8 percent; her lifetime risk calculated by the Gail model was 17.1 percent. But Gail didn't factor in her breast density, height and weight, or menopausal status, or her mother's breast cancers.

In our practice, we most commonly use the Tyrer-Cuzick model to assess risk for our patients, since it's the most comprehensive. But it's important to note that we assess patients using both the Tyrer-Cuzick and Gail models and use the highest score to determine which patients should have increased surveillance with MRIs, consider taking tamoxifen or an aromatase inhibitor for risk reduction, or consider preventive surgery. The reason that there are a number of different risk assessment models is because none are perfect; until we find the optimal risk assessment tools, various providers will choose the model that they're most comfortable with or that provides the highest risk result to offer the most careful approach for their patients. Some providers prefer Tyrer-Cuzick, while others prefer the Gail model; but both are excellent, albeit imperfect, tools to help stratify a woman's risk for developing breast cancer in the next five years, and over their lifetime.

Currently, risk assessment tools are based on population information; that is, how often women with risks like yours develop breast cancer. However, new assessment tools are currently being developed that use the enormous amount of individualized information (also called proteomic information) in *your* mammogram to calculate your risk, not population data. When that tool is made available, it will reflect your own personal risk instead of your risk relative to the population. Screen-Point Medical, a Norwegian company, is using FDA-approved artificial intelligence to augment the enormous amount of personal information based on the character and type of breast tissue in your own mammogram to improve breast cancer diagnosis on mammograms. This development will include all the factors evaluated in the other assessment tools, as well as the proteomic information in your mammogram to more accurately determine your risk. It can be frustrating that the three risk models we rely on can give such markedly different results, and we look forward to harnessing the proteomic information in a woman's mammogram or other imaging to assess her *specific* risk, not her risk based on population information. This technology should be in clinical use soon.

HOW TO REDUCE YOUR RISK

Women with an increased risk of breast cancer are often plagued by their fear of getting breast cancer. Many have stood by family members who were suffering through the process of diagnosis, treatment, and, in some cases, a losing battle with breast cancer. What they want to do above all else is avoid a similar fate themselves, and spare their loved ones from the experience, too.

If you're impacted by any of the conditions that increase your likelihood of getting breast cancer, what can be done?

Leading a healthy lifestyle with a diet of fresh fruits and vegetables accompanied with regular exercise can decrease the risk, of course, but it may not be enough to significantly move the needle from high risk to low. And remember, even women who live arguably the healthiest lifestyles are not spared from getting breast cancer, since 75 percent of women with breast cancer have no risk factors other than being a woman.

In women at substantially increased risk, careful screening with scans every six months is the standard protocol designed to find cancer early, when it can be eradicated with better results, but it doesn't reduce your risk of breast cancer. While many women take these scans in stride, grateful to have an early-warning system in place, the idea of constant surveillance or screening—sometimes accompanied by additional imaging and biopsies—can feel challenging or even unacceptable.

For those women, the years of anxious anticipation surrounding each test can be obviated by removing their healthy breasts. Yes, this is somewhat radical. While most women will understandably choose to keep their breasts, for some women with a very high risk of breast cancer or with a previous diagnosis of breast cancer, consideration of bilateral preventive mastectomies is very reasonable. In fact, it's no longer radical. In women diagnosed with breast cancer, never having to worry about getting cancer in the opposite breast, even if it's unlikely to happen, can be a profound relief.[21] There is a way to change the narrative; instead of diagnosing breast cancer early, breast cancer can be prevented with preventive or prophylactic mastectomies.

It isn't a decision to be taken lightly, but it is an important option to consider. It's the one we both chose. Many of our patients have as well. In our experience, it's extremely rare to hear that a patient who has undergone preventive mastectomies regrets her decision, even if she misses her natural breasts. Most women feel that an enormous weight has been lifted from their minds.

When genetic testing showed that our patient Carrie Thomas and her sister didn't have the BRCA mutation, they were both relieved. Their mother had been diagnosed with breast cancer at thirty-three and again in her forties. After her second diagnosis, she had bilateral mastectomies without reconstruction, long before genetic testing was even available. She had testing done at the same time her daughters did, and the results showed that she didn't have a genetic mutation, either. But despite a negative test, the history of breast cancer in both breasts at a young age was a significant and concerning indication that she might have a genetic mutation that researchers have not yet found.

We treated Carrie and her sister as if they could have a mutation since their mother also tested negative. Neither was interested in having preventive mastectomies. They were happy with the surveillance of MRIs between their annual mammograms. But when Carrie's sister was found to have an early breast cancer at age forty, Carrie decided her own risk was too great and opted for preventive mastectomies. When her sister was diagnosed with breast cancer, she had bilateral nipple-sparing mastectomies with implant reconstructions. Carrie was relieved to see how happy her sister was with the results. Since Carrie's surgery was elective, she was able to choose the best time to fit it into her personal and work life. While she doesn't feel that the results are perfect, since there's some rippling of the implants and they don't feel like her natural breasts did, she knows that the decision was the right one for her, and she was happy to have control of the timing of her surgery.

Studies confirm that preventive mastectomies give the same advantage to women with an increased risk for breast cancer or strong family history as they do to women with a genetic mutation. Electively removing healthy breasts reduces the risk of cancer by 90 to 95 percent.[22] This gives a woman previously at markedly increased risk for breast cancer a risk that's lower, closer to 1 to 2 percent, than the average woman, who has a 12 percent lifetime risk.

Between 2003 and 2010, the percentage of women under forty-five undergoing preventive mastectomies *tripled* (from 9.3 percent to 26.4 percent) in the United States.[23] If their surgeon makes no recommendation for or against it, women tend to choose preventive mastectomies on their own.[24] When they discuss it with a *female* surgeon, women are three times more likely to choose preventive mastectomy.[25] Eighty-two percent of women who opt for preventive mastectomies say they want to avoid worrying about a recurrence of cancer.[26] The experiences of close friends and family who have had breast cancer treatments also influence their choices.[27] Women who place a high value on being in control of their own treatment are the most likely to consider double mastectomies, while those who consider themselves to be logical are less likely to make that choice.[28]

Though it may sound like we're strongly recommending preventive mastectomies, we aren't. It isn't the right decision for everyone. Most women prefer to keep their breasts and are comfortable with surveillance. That's an excellent decision, since we have so many imaging options available. Women at high risk for breast cancer who choose surveillance, *if* diagnosed with breast cancer, are extremely likely to be diagnosed at an early and treatable stage. But keep in mind that once you have breast cancer, there will likely be additional treatments. The only way to reduce your risk of needing those treatments is to avoid getting breast cancer altogether.

With that in mind, as soon as Rachel learned that she was indeed BRCA1 positive, she scheduled preventive mastectomies for herself. At the time, Rachel was the director of the Breast Imaging Section at the Johns Hopkins Medical Institutions, and as such was charged with deciding what equipment to purchase for the center. Between scheduling her preventive mastectomies, while trying out new ultrasound equipment on herself to assess image quality, she unexpectedly found her own breast cancer. What was to be preventive ended up being breast cancer treatment when her breast cancer was diagnosed. She had bilateral mastectomies and underwent chemotherapy. Rachel had hoped to prevent ever getting breast cancer, but timing was not on her side. This demonstrates that women at markedly increased risk of breast cancer can choose the time for their preventive mastectomy, but their risk remains high, and cancer can occur at any time. We've seen too many patients in our practice who know they will eventually undergo preventive mastectomies but whose plans are changed when cancer is diagnosed before the time they choose to have those mastectomies. This is also something to consider—yes, you can choose the time to undergo preventive mastectomies, but there's no guarantee that cancer won't develop while you wait. This doesn't mean you can't schedule preventive mastectomies to optimally suit your schedule. You certainly can, and it will usually work out. But in women with markedly increased risk of breast cancer—indeed, in all women—cancer comes in its own time, not ours.

Christy was able to take action and essentially guarantee that she would not be diagnosed with the cancer that took her mother's life. We both chose to have mastectomies and would do it again. We support any women considering the option, but we also strongly support and carefully care for those women who choose surveillance. There is no right or wrong decision.

Common Questions to Discuss with Your Care Team

What tool do you use to determine my risk for breast cancer?

What other risk tools are there, and how do they change my risk of breast cancer?

What is my five-year and lifetime risk for breast cancer?

Do you recommend that I have MRIs in addition to mammograms?

Is there any other screening that I might need because of my breast density or family history?

How do I know whether I have dense breasts?

What does having dense breasts mean in terms of my risk of breast cancer? Are there any additional screenings I might benefit from?

What is atypical hyperplasia, and what does that mean for me?

What is lobular carcinoma in situ, and what does that mean for me?

Should I consider prophylactic mastectomies, and if so, why?

What can I do to reduce my risk?

How can I find out if I have a genetic mutation that increases my risk of breast cancer?

If I do have a genetic mutation that increases my risk of breast cancer, what is my risk, and what other cancers am I at risk for?

Should I see a genetic counselor?

CHAPTER 6

You Have Breast Cancer at a Young Age

Jocelyn Clarke's wedding was only four months away when she got the news. She had just booked the perfect venue: a holiday resort on the cliffs overlooking the Atlantic. Friends and relatives were already saying how eager they were to come. The last thing Jocelyn wanted to think about was any kind of medical issue, much less triple-negative breast cancer. She was only twenty-nine.

Life was perfect for Jocelyn. She was excited about her upcoming marriage, and had recently been promoted to a new position at work, a job that she loved. But one day when she was in the shower, she noted a mass in her left breast. Rachel performed an ultrasound, which showed a suspicious mass, and subsequently did a mammogram as well. Jocelyn had a needle biopsy done that same day, which confirmed that it was a cancer. When we told her the diagnosis, she could hardly believe it. Breast cancer is rare in women under forty. There was no history of breast cancer in her family. Her genetic testing showed that she didn't have a BRCA mutation. It was understandably a shock.

Because her type of breast cancer was aggressive, we started neoadjuvant chemotherapy (chemotherapy before surgery) right away. It was a struggle, but in the months before her marriage, she managed to work in wedding planning around the regular treatments. When her hair started falling out, her heart sank. She knew it would likely happen, but she had already imagined herself with a wedding hairstyle that complemented her gown, a crushing loss. When her fiancé reminded her how much he wanted to marry her and how little he cared about her hair, Jocelyn rallied. Instead of wearing a wig, she walked down the aisle on her wedding day in a beautiful dress with her bald head proudly held high.

After her honeymoon, she returned to schedule surgery. She wanted to remove both her breasts even though she had the option of conserving her affected breast. The experience of chemotherapy had made the decision easy for her: she never wanted to go through that again. What she did enjoy was picking out the size and shape of her implants for reconstruction. She found the surgery to be much easier than the chemotherapy and appreciated the required time off from work. Jocelyn loves her new breasts, and her new husband does, too. And the greatest news was that there was no sign of residual cancer in the final pathology, which meant the chemotherapy worked!

LOOKING FOR EARLY CANCER

Even when the outcome is as positive as it was for Jocelyn, a diagnosis of cancer is always a challenge. It's especially hard for young women who are single, married and want to have children, or eager to pursue a successful career. At a time when women should look optimistically toward the future, cancer puts on the brakes and forces them to face their fears about fertility, children, intimacy, finances, career, and, of course, survival.

Unfortunately, young women often get a type of breast cancer that's more aggressive than the cancers in older women, which results in lower chances of survival.[1] In some ways, it isn't even the same cancer. Breast cancer in young women differs biologically from breast cancer in older women in that it's more frequently triple-negative, a type of breast cancer with a worse prognosis.[2] While breast cancer in younger women is rare, it's still the most common cancer among women ages fifteen to thirty-nine. An astonishing fact is that 5 percent of all breast cancers are diagnosed in women under forty; that's nearly fifteen thousand cases per year in the United States.[3] Overall, about 11 percent of all breast cancers occur in women younger than forty-five, according to the Centers for Disease Control and Prevention (CDC). An estimated 26,393 women under forty-five are expected to be diagnosed with breast cancer in 2022.

So how can women under the age of forty find their breast cancer, especially when screening mammography in average-risk women doesn't begin until age forty? They need to empower themselves with a clear understanding of their breasts, with monthly self-examination, so that if anything changes, they are aware. Anytime a woman feels a breast mass—either while doing a breast self-exam or incidentally—that doesn't go away, she should get it checked out. This is true for women of any age. Even if a woman feels something concerning in her breast and has a normal mammogram, that's not a guarantee that she doesn't have breast cancer. Women can have breast cancer that isn't seen on a mammogram but that may be detected by physical examination, ultrasound, or MRI. In fact, mammograms are not as effective in women with dense breast tissue, the kind of breast tissue an overwhelming majority of young women have. As a result, when cancer is discovered, it has often had time to develop to a later stage.[4] An increasing number of young women are being diagnosed with metastatic breast cancer, breast cancer that has spread to other organs.[5]

Almost 80 percent of young women with breast cancer find it themselves and ask their doctors about it.[6] Doing so can save your life. Be vigilant about a lump in your breasts, but remember that a lump isn't the only sign of cancer. Any abnormality, such as a change in the shape of your breast or discharge from a nipple, should raise a red flag. Too many women dismiss the signs because they assume they're too young to have cancer.[7] In fact, more than one thousand women under forty die of breast cancer every year.[8] Early detection is critical in avoiding this outcome.

Young women sometimes feel a mass in their breasts during their menstrual cycles. That's normal, and should resolve in one or two menstrual cycles. If it doesn't, or if you feel something suspicious in your breasts, it's critical that you have it checked out, even if you've been assured by your healthcare provider that it's nothing. If the area of concern persists for several months, make certain that it's evaluated by your healthcare provider and that imaging, such as a mammogram and/or an ultrasound, is obtained. Often, when young women feel a mass in their breast, the initial imaging is an ultrasound, because frequently the lump can be identified as a simple cyst that needs no further evaluation. However, it has to be determined that it isn't cancer. One thing young women should *not* do is accept that it's "nothing"; if you remain concerned after seeing a doctor, see another doctor or a surgeon who specializes in patients with breast issues. You must advocate for yourself. You must be persistent. If your concerns are dismissed as nothing or you're told it's a cyst without the imaging confirmation that this is true, be dogged in getting the imaging you need to confirm that it is actually "nothing." Most of the time, it will indeed be nothing. But the continued self-advocacy might well save your life. Unfortunately, we've seen so many young women who were concerned about something in their breasts but were assured that they were too young to get breast cancer, only to subsequently be diagnosed with late-stage cancer. You are your own best advocate. Advocating for yourself can save your life.

With the increasing use of in vitro fertilization, many young women ask if having IVF increases their chance of breast cancer. Although initially there was some thought that it might, the scientific evidence indicates that IVF doesn't increase a woman's chance of breast cancer.[9]

Age alone doesn't change the treatment for breast cancer. The stage of the cancer, its tumor grade, and its characteristics (hormone receptor and HER2 status) are more likely to determine the type of treatment a doctor recommends. Younger women may be more inclined to choose breast reconstruction after a mastectomy than older women, who may prefer the simplest, safest, least invasive option. Breast conservation is always a reasonable consideration for those who are candidates for it. Studies have shown that the risk of a local recurrence in patients with a genetic mutation is similar in those without a mutation,[10] but the lifetime risk of developing another cancer in the other breast can be as high as 55 percent.[11] In fact, the age that a woman is diagnosed with breast cancer impacts her likelihood of developing another breast cancer. Women who are diagnosed with breast cancer have a 0.5 to 1.0 percent per year risk of a new cancer in either breast. Therefore, if a woman is diagnosed at forty years old and lives to eighty, her risk of a new cancer can be as high as 20 to 40 percent by the end of her life, compared to 12 percent for an eighty-year-old woman without a personal history.[12]

Studies have shown that the risk of dying of breast cancer doesn't change whether you choose to have a mastectomy initially or have a lumpectomy first and, if you have a subsequent recurrence, have a mastectomy. Although the outcome is the same, keep in mind that treatment for a second breast cancer may be more difficult. Overall, young women are more likely to choose to have bilateral mastectomies even if they don't have a known mutation.[13]

When it comes to making decisions about treatment, it's important to keep in in mind the factors that impact young women diagnosed with breast cancer. We see women who are single and dating, have young children at home, or lack flexibility at work. We hear their concerns about gaining weight, losing their hair, experiencing decreased libido, or becoming menopausal due to chemotherapy or surgery. They may be more concerned about how the treatments will affect their body image and their experience of intimacy. If they're pregnant, the treatment becomes complicated, because the issue is not only treating the cancer but protecting the baby. These are all very critical considerations that affect young women facing a diagnosis of breast cancer. It's important to have a medical team that understands the concerns that face each patient, so if you're under forty and have been diagnosed with breast cancer, be sure to talk through all your lifestyle factors with your doctors to fully understand how treatment options will impact you. Make certain you find a doctor and a team that listens to your concerns and with whom you're comfortable talking about the medical and nonmedical-but-critical issues regarding your diagnosis and treatment.

It's important to know that you have some time to find the right team for you. That being said, time remains critical, and you shouldn't be paralyzed by the need to choose a team. Prioritize finding a team that cares for a large number of breast cancer patients. In fact, it's best if your team specializes in breast problems. There are many medical teams specializing exclusively in breast issues for patients of all ages and backgrounds. Having a team dedicated to treating women with breast cancer can offer many critical resources, including support groups to help you through these times. The care of all women with breast cancer, including young women, involves a comprehensive approach to address the numerous needs women have and the issues they face. Be sure to mention to your care team what other health needs and priorities you have. These full-picture conversations are critically important.

BREAST CANCER TREATMENT AND FERTILITY

While only 5 percent of breast cancer occurs in women under the age of forty, there are still over eleven thousand cases per year in the United States. Breast cancer is now the most common cancer in women under the age of forty and in women who are either pregnant or have recently had a baby.[14]

In women of childbearing age, discussion of chemotherapy can raise questions about preserving fertility or causing early menopause. We want to be clear about the factors at play here.

Chemotherapy can cause damage to the ovaries, induce irregular periods, or cause monthly periods to stop, bringing on early menopause.[15] If you were planning to have children, this issue must be addressed and considered prior to beginning treatment. Once diagnosed with breast cancer, there's a necessary delay of at least two years before you can try to become pregnant.

For most young women, periods will return following chemotherapy. But because chemotherapy treatment can make it more difficult to have children and significantly shorten the window of time for getting pregnant, it's important to understand and carefully consider the options for fertility preservation. After taking tamoxifen, a women's periods usually resume, but they can be sporadic. The general recommendation for women taking tamoxifen as part of their treatment is to continue tamoxifen for five to ten years. However, since it must be stopped prior to attempting to get pregnant, it can be given for as few as two to three years for those who wish to become pregnant. Fertility normally declines with every year as we get older, and this decline can hasten following chemotherapy. It's important to know that there's a danger of birth defects if a woman becomes pregnant while she's taking tamoxifen.[16] It must be discontinued several months before trying to become pregnant. Another important consideration for young women discussing mastectomies is that they won't be able to nurse their children. While it might seem overwhelming to be considering fertility issues right after a breast cancer diagnosis, it's important that you do, since the decisions you make about treatment can have an irreversible impact on your fertility. Similarly, different drugs may be chosen as a result of fertility considerations. That's why it's so important to consider these issues at a time when so many other treatment decisions are being made.

Amanda Young took tamoxifen as part of her treatment when she was diagnosed with breast cancer at the age of twenty-six because her tumor was estrogen-receptor-positive (ER-positive). She wasn't married at the time, but knew she wanted to have and nurse children, so even though she had the BRCA2 mutation, she chose not to have mastectomies. After having breast-conservation surgery, Amanda underwent chemotherapy, followed by radiation to her affected breast.

A few years later, at twenty-nine, Amanda got married. When she was ready to try to get pregnant, she stopped the tamoxifen, and was able to have two healthy children. She couldn't nurse them from the breast that had been treated with radiation, since radiation prevents milk production, but she was able to nurse from the unaffected breast. She waited until her children were slightly older to have bilateral mastectomies with reconstruction, and is planning on having her ovaries removed when she's in her forties.

For women over the age of thirty-five, chemotherapy increases the risk of entering menopause and, therefore, no longer being able to have children. Because chemotherapy attacks all fast-growing cells, it can destroy healthy cells anywhere in the body, including the ovaries. Some studies have shown that drugs such as goserelin (Zoladex), leuprorelin (Lupron), and triptorelin may be able to protect the ovaries during chemotherapy by shutting them down, which can reduce the odds of early menopause as well as protect fertility.[17] If you're going to undergo chemotherapy and want to preserve fertility, a discussion with your doctor as well as a doctor specializing in fertility is warranted.

One of the best ways to preserve fertility is to have your eggs frozen before starting chemotherapy. In most cases, you will be able to briefly delay your treatment while the eggs are collected and stored without affecting your prognosis.[18] Because fertility preservation generally only delays treatment by a few weeks, it's considered safe. The good news is that the chance of having a successful pregnancy after freezing your eggs is now similar to IVF with embryos, which means that single women who don't have a partner also have the opportunity to freeze their eggs. The egg can be fertilized in the future, when the woman chooses. In most cases, your odds of getting pregnant from a previously frozen egg are 30 to 60 percent. Eggs can be harvested whether they're fertilized or not, before you start chemotherapy treatment. When you're ready, they can be thawed and fertilized in the lab with an intracytoplasmic sperm injection (ICSI), where one healthy sperm is injected directly into the egg.[19]

Studies have now clearly demonstrated that the medications used for ovarian stimulation to preserve eggs don't have any adverse effects on patients' breast cancer survival rates. It's also important to know that no studies have demonstrated an increased risk of breast cancer recurrence in women who become pregnant after completing treatment.

Our patient Amy Thompson was diagnosed with breast cancer at thirty-two, not long after she got married. She and her new husband both wanted to have children. Since her tumor was HER2 positive, it was important for her to undergo chemotherapy, but we could safely wait several weeks while she completed the fertility-preservation process. She went through fertility treatments and had embryos frozen before she began chemotherapy.

Two years after she completed radiation and a year after taking Herceptin, she got pregnant using her embryos and delivered a beautiful girl. When she was first diagnosed with breast cancer, she had considered the option of having mastectomies, but chose to keep her breasts since she was newly married at the time of diagnosis, and it was even more important to her that she be able to breastfeed children. She knows that she can have mastectomies in the future if that's the direction she chooses.

If you want to have children after breast cancer treatment, it's a good idea to discuss the latest fertility-preservation options with a fertility specialist in addition to your breast surgeon and oncologist. We recommend seeing a specialist as soon as you learn of your diagnosis so that if you choose fertility preservation, those treatments can begin right away and avoid delaying surgery or chemotherapy by more than a few weeks.

BREAST CANCER AND PREGNANCY

For new mothers and pregnant women, breast cancer is the most common form of cancer, occurring in one out of every three thousand pregnancies.[20] Almost one-third of all breast cancer diagnoses in young women are made in the first years after the birth of a child.[21]

It was remarkably bad timing when Patrice found out she was pregnant just after she was diagnosed with HER2-positive breast cancer at the age of twenty-nine. Since she was early in the first trimester, we sadly recommended that she terminate the pregnancy so that we could start chemotherapy treatment with Herceptin. This is a devastating conversation to have, but it's important for patients and physicians to be able to discuss all the factors and possible options in a health crisis. Herceptin is a lifesaving medication, but it cannot be given at any time during pregnancy, nor can the chemotherapy that's normally given with it. We needed to be clear with Patrice about all the options available, and ensure that we, doctor and patient, were on the same page.

Patrice chose to keep the baby. She had a mastectomy with implant reconstruction in the beginning of her second trimester, and was then treated with a form of chemotherapy known to be safe during pregnancy. After she delivered, she was treated with Herceptin and Taxol. She subsequently decided to have the other breast removed, mostly for symmetry, since it became so large during pregnancy, but also because she didn't want to have to worry about a new cancer in the future. She has no regrets. She has a beautiful daughter named Angel, and is grateful every day.

Eliminating cancer is the goal, whether or not a woman is pregnant, but protecting the fetus takes additional precautions. Overall breast cancer outcomes are about the same whether a woman is pregnant or not, but pregnancy can make breast cancer harder to diagnose and treat. Some oncologists say that the spread of the cancer can be slowed by ending a pregnancy, but not everyone agrees. It makes the treatment less complex, but there's no solid evidence that terminating a pregnancy improves the outcome of breast cancer, and there are no studies proving that breast cancer harms the fetus.[22] Termination is generally only recommended when the diagnosis of breast cancer is made early in the first trimester, often before the woman even knows she's pregnant.

Treatments during pregnancy will be governed primarily by the size and location of the tumor, the duration of the pregnancy, and the health of the mother. Most doctors feel that certain chemotherapy drugs, namely those that don't cross the placenta and therefore cannot access the fetus, are safe in the second and third trimester of pregnancy. However, hormone therapy, targeted therapy, and radiation therapy are too dangerous during pregnancy.[23] Generally, we try not to have a woman undergo surgery during the first trimester of pregnancy due to the potential harm of anesthesia and surgery at a time when the fetus's organs are developing. The first trimester is in many ways the most critical to birth defects. While it's considered safe to have breast cancer surgery after the first trimester, certain other treatments cannot be given until after delivery due to the harm they can cause to the developing baby, although some chemotherapies can.

Women who are diagnosed with breast cancer shortly after having a baby are generally advised to stop breastfeeding during cancer treatment. This helps reduce the flow of blood to the breasts, which makes them smaller. Not only does this help during surgery, it can also reduce the risk of infection or milk fistula, where milk might leak from the surgical incision. More concerning is that chemotherapy drugs can be passed on to the baby in the breast milk, so continuing to breastfeed during chemotherapy, hormone therapy, or targeted therapy is not recommended.[24]

When Donna Simpson was diagnosed with an early-stage HER2-positive breast cancer at the age of thirty-two, she was thirty-six weeks pregnant. Her breasts were much larger and denser than normal, but she was concerned about how different they seemed; she had felt changes in her right breast that were different from the left. An ultrasound showed a large mass concerning for cancer, and ultrasound-guided needle biopsy confirmed the diagnosis. The safest option was to induce delivery of her baby early the following week; she was far enough along in her pregnancy that we were confident the baby would be fine, and doing this meant she could start chemotherapy and Herceptin. She had an excellent response to both. She was disappointed that she couldn't breastfeed her child, but relieved to learn that the baby would be protected from the cancer treatments. She also appreciated that others could bottle-feed her daughter when she was not feeling well after her treatments. Her mother loved feeding her new grandchild!

Once Donna finished chemotherapy, she knew that mastectomies were the right option for her, even though her genetic testing results were negative for mutations. She really wanted to keep her nipples, so we recommended a combined staging procedure that included a breast reduction performed by a plastic surgeon when Christy performed a partial mastectomy and sentinel lymph node biopsy. Several months later, Donna had nipple-sparing mastectomies with reconstructions using her abdominal fat. She's thrilled with how her new breasts look, and loves that she no longer has the extra abdominal fat that she developed during pregnancy. Donna is relieved that she had bilateral mastectomies to obviate the risk of breast cancer in her other breast.

Final Thoughts

It's a lot of information to take in all at once. Give yourself time to reflect on it and talk it over with loved ones. Don't feel you have to decide immediately. Even with a cancer diagnosis, you have the time to carefully consider your options. Days and weeks won't change your outcome, and youth gives you the advantage of time.

It's important to understand the pros and cons of any treatment your doctor recommends. Be sure to ask how it will affect your quality of life and whether it will extend your life.[25] While your doctor may recommend that you keep your breasts and undergo surveillance, you may prefer to have preventive mastectomies. Participate actively in the decision-making process, which may include research on your own and discussion with others besides your surgeon. If you aren't comfortable with the recommendations you're given, get a second opinion, or a third. Your surgeon won't have to live with the consequences—you will. Only when you know your options can you decide which one is right for you.

MASTECTOMIES IN YOUNG WOMEN

Regardless of your fertility or pregnancy status, it's a big decision to have bilateral mastectomies, whether you have a cancer diagnosis and/or a known genetic mutation or not. Having a genetic mutation makes the decision more straightforward than for young women who test negative, because the data is clearer.

Everyone asks, "If I need a mastectomy on the breast with cancer, should I have the other breast removed even if I don't have a genetic mutation?" Or, "If I do have a genetic mutation but am a candidate for breast conservation, do I have the option of keeping my breasts?" The answer is yes to both these questions. Again, different decisions are correct for different people. However, it's important to remember that once you have breast cancer, even if you have bilateral mastectomies, you aren't guaranteed that the cancer won't return. It's the best way to minimize that risk, but it isn't a guarantee.

Breast reconstruction often requires multiple surgeries. Going in and out of anesthesia and surgery, with all that entails, the entire process can take up to a year.

The cosmetic results can be excellent following reconstruction, but reconstructed breasts are not native breasts. Nipple and breast sensation will be mostly or completely gone. Even if the new breasts look better than the original ones, they're not the same. On the other hand, there are also issues with keeping your breasts. You will need to have ongoing imaging, likely consisting of mammograms alternating with MRIs every six months. You may need a biopsy, or even more than one. And worst of all, the biopsy results may show breast cancer. The decision is very personal when breast conservation is an option, and only you can decide what is best for you.

In the medical literature, you'll find studies that run the gamut of satisfied women or dissatisfied women who have made either decision—that is, mastectomy or lumpectomy (partial mastectomy). It's important to realize that how satisfied a woman is depends on many factors—these differ for each woman and include things like how pleased she is with the cosmetic outcome, what her expectations were, where and what her support network is like, and, of course, what her prognosis is. There are so many variables that it's hard to pinpoint exactly why different women feel as they do. Every woman's outcome and experience is different. Nevertheless, what is important is to realize that there are satisfied and dissatisfied women who have made both choices. There is no single correct decision, since there's no perfect solution to this difficult issue.

In one study women with breast conservation reported a slightly higher quality of life than women with one or both breasts removed. Their satisfaction with their breasts, as well as their psychosocial and sexual well-being, were higher, but curiously enough, they felt their physical well-being was not.[26] More than one study has shown that women who had nipple-sparing mastectomies were less satisfied with sexual intimacy because of the notable lack of sensation in their nipples and breasts.[27] For some women, feeling and sensation can improve over time, but it's rare for women to regain the sensation they felt before surgery.

Over the past several years, mastectomies in young women have gone up almost tenfold. Laura Dominici, MD, FACS, a surgeon at the Dana-Farber Brigham Cancer Center and assistant professor of surgery at Harvard Medical School, conducted a study to find out whether the women who underwent preventive mastectomies were actually achieving what they wanted.

Many studies provided data about the oncological outcomes or life spans, but Dr. Dominici wondered about their subjective experiences. Were they happier? Did they feel better? How did they feel about their breasts afterward?[28]

Dr. Ann Partridge, Dr. Dominici's colleague at Dana-Farber, had already followed a group of young women diagnosed with breast cancer from 2006 to 2016. "So, it was really the right population," Dr. Dominici said. "And these women have been wonderful participants . . . a nice group of women who were agreeable to fill out surveys and also for whom we had an opportunity to have very long-term follow-up." The survey questions asked about each woman's satisfaction with her breasts, her sexual well-being, and emotional issues such as anxiety, depression, and happiness.[29] What they found was that women who chose bilateral mastectomy were more likely to be younger and had higher psychosocial and breast satisfaction than those who did not, but that their physical well-being was lower. But perhaps most significantly, they concluded that the magnitude of the difference between the two groups was too small to be clinically meaningful. There isn't a huge difference in the happiness and psychosocial well-being between those who did undergo prophylactic mastectomy on the other breast and those who did not.

The decision about which surgical option is best for you is very personal. Data shows that survival outcomes are equal with lumpectomy and mastectomy, but the considerations that accompany each decision are different. These decisions can be particularly difficult since they aren't based on a known outcome. Women are asked to make an irreversible decision at a particularly difficult and emotional time in their lives. Therefore, it's important to have thorough discussions with your doctors and those who support you, not only about the cancer considerations but about things like how you will look and feel, as well as what the follow-up considerations are. All aspects of the cancer diagnosis, if you had one, and the surgical choices are important and require careful consideration.

When we talk to our patients, we tell them candidly that the benefits of preventive mastectomies seem to be greater in younger women diagnosed with breast cancer, particularly in those with a genetic mutation. For a thirty-year-old woman who has a BRCA1 or BRCA2 mutation, a preventive mastectomy may add three to five years to her life. For a woman above age sixty, the gain in life span is smaller.[30]

Tonya Henry was diagnosed with an ER-positive HER2-negative breast cancer when she was thirty-five years old. Since the tumor was large relative to her breast size, we recommended a mastectomy. She was very thin, with unusually low body fat, so her only option was implant reconstruction. She could have had only the affected breast removed, but it would have meant the reconstructed breast would not be symmetrical to her native breast. She didn't like the idea of mismatched breasts and didn't want to worry about getting cancer in the other breast in the future, so she elected to have bilateral nipple-sparing mastectomies.

When she heard that we could make her breasts larger if we did expander reconstructions, she saw a silver lining. Her breasts had always been smaller than what she hoped, so she opted for expanders. We put them in before chemotherapy, and when that treatment was complete, the expanders were replaced with permanent implants. She's happy with her somewhat larger breasts, and is also pleased that she no longer needs careful surveillance with imaging. She also appreciates the increased security of a lower risk of developing a new cancer.

Many young women diagnosed with breast cancer decide that the time isn't right for preventive mastectomies, knowing that they can always do it later. Insurance will still pay for it, as long as the doctors agree. Some women who initially had breast conservation surgery for breast cancer ultimately choose to have mastectomies after being treated with chemotherapy.

It's reassuring to know that most women's partners and families support their decision to have preventive mastectomies. The main concern for women and their loved ones is that they do everything they can to optimize their chance of survival. When counseling patients about mastectomies, we discuss the cosmetic aspect of the surgery quite a lot. As we discuss in chapter 9, reconstructed breasts are a woman's "new normal." Our plastic surgeons do everything possible to make the reconstructed breasts look as beautiful as they can. But we, and those we care for, never forget that the ultimate goal is to achieve a long and healthy life. Plastic surgeons are now working on techniques to improve sensation for women undergoing reconstruction to further improve patient satisfaction, although we aren't there yet.[31]

Even with enormous love and support from your family and friends, it's a difficult decision. It's important to be honest about the fact that, while there are good things about preventive mastectomies, there are downsides, too.

For couples, mourning the loss of their mutual sexual experience around the woman's breasts is understandable. While it's a small thing in the context of life and death, it's a loss nonetheless. Going through the pros and cons as candidly as possible can bring a couple closer. While partners ordinarily find women just as sexually attractive after breast reconstruction as before, there's always an adjustment as women become accustomed to their new, reconstructed breasts.[32] This is discussed in more detail in chapter 10.

Women are increasingly choosing to undergo bilateral prophylactic mastectomy even when early breast cancer is diagnosed in just one breast. In the 1990s, approximately 5 percent of women underwent a contralateral prophylactic mastectomy. Now that figure is between 11 and 25 percent, a significant increase. There's no specific data about why this is, but it has been a continuing trend. Perhaps it's because nipple-sparing mastectomies are now an option and cosmetic results continue to improve; maybe it's because there's now data on how effective prophylactic mastectomy is; or maybe it's because prophylactic mastectomy has become far more accepted. It's also possible that all the recent data about the increased risk of a second cancer in the other breast is influencing more women's decisions. As a result of the marked increase in the procedure, researchers at Duke University wondered whether women who chose bilateral mastectomies had a better quality of life. They found that women who had contralateral prophylactic mastectomy reported slightly higher psychosocial well-being—feeling confident, emotionally healthy, and accepting of their bodies. However, the differences between women who underwent prophylactic mastectomy on the healthy breast and those who did not were very small and diminished over time. Psychosocial well-being continued to increase in both groups, even ten years after treatment.[33]

The reality is that every patient's outcome varies. Even when women undergo the same treatments, their reactions to those treatments will differ. But that makes it all that much more important for you to be as well-informed as possible and have realistic expectations about the long-term results of treatment and surgery. You have the opportunity to potentially change your future with mastectomies and reduce your concern about getting another breast cancer, albeit at a very significant cost to your body, your emotions, and your family. Yes, it can be difficult to make such consequential decisions, especially while you're feeling emotional and even afraid, but we hope we've shared information that can help you make the right decision for yourself.

Common Questions to Discuss
with Your Care Team

Am I more at risk for having another breast cancer if my mother and/or sister have it, even if our genetic testing is negative?

What is the five-year survival rate for someone my age?

Is it possible that, after treatment, the breast cancer will never return?

How will treatment affect my fertility?

Should I take the precaution of freezing my eggs beforehand?

Will it be safe for me to have children after treatment?

Am I more likely to need aggressive chemo because I'm young?

What should I expect, and how will I feel during chemotherapy?

Will my age help me recover from the side effects of the treatment?

Will I be able to work during chemo?

Does chemo cause early menopause? If so, is there a way to decrease the chances of it happening?

How long do I need to take Tamoxifen if I want to become pregnant in the next year or two?

Will Tamoxifen trigger menopause?

Do you have any support groups for women my age?

How do I tell my children about my diagnosis and treatment?

If I keep my breasts, what will my follow-up be?

If I have mastectomies, what will my follow-up be?

If I need a mastectomy on the cancer side, should I consider having a mastectomy on the healthy side? Do I have the option of having the healthy breast removed if that's my preference?

If I have the option of breast conservation, do I still have the option of bilateral mastectomies?

What about immunotherapy or clinical trials? Are any appropriate for me, and should I consider either of these options?

CHAPTER 7

You Have Postmenopausal Breast Cancer

As if the hot flashes, night sweats, volatile emotions, and brain fog weren't enough, now you're diagnosed with cancer?! Menopause doesn't cause breast cancer, but getting older does increase the risk of getting it. Most breast cancers occur in postmenopausal women over the age of fifty-five years. In fact, *two-thirds* of all new breast cancer diagnoses occur in postmenopausal women.[1] The good news is that breast cancer in older women often grows slowly and has characteristics that help with more targeted treatment. When breast cancer is diagnosed early, a woman who receives the appropriate treatment tends to have a better outcome than a younger woman who generally has a more aggressive cancer.[2]

In the United States, the median age of women diagnosed with breast cancer is sixty-two. The risk of breast cancer increases with each year of life.[3] Other than being a woman, which is the greatest risk for breast cancer, age is the next most important risk factor. The older you are, the greater your risk. That's why the risk of getting breast cancer increases after menopause. But age alone isn't the only risk factor. Other risk factors include greater cumulative estrogen exposure.

Women with early menstruation (before age twelve) and late menopause (after age fifty-five) have an increased breast cancer risk. Estrogen stimulates the uterus and breast tissue during menstruation. The more periods a woman has, the more her body has been exposed to estrogen.[4] It's this awareness that first raised questions about the safety and potential breast cancer risk of the use of hormonal replacement therapy (HRT) as a treatment for menopausal symptoms. We now know that the use of HRT after menopause, even bioequivalent HRT, does increase the risk of breast cancer. While initial studies tested therapies that combined estrogen and progestin, it's possible that there's an even higher risk in women taking HRT consisting of estrogen alone.[5] It's now widely accepted that there's a direct correlation between HRT and breast cancer. For some women, the benefits of taking HRT outweigh the risks.[6] However, we strongly encourage our patients not to take HRT due to the increased risk of breast cancer. If you're taking HRT and are diagnosed with breast cancer, you will need to stop taking it.

There are ways to deal with the symptoms of menopause without the use of hormone replacements. These include regular exercise, reducing stress, getting eight hours of sleep every night, quitting smoking, and avoiding hot flash triggers like coffee, tea, and alcohol. Lifestyle changes can be very effective. For example, some women notice that if they drink coffee before they shower, they experience significant hot flashes, but not if they drink coffee after they shower. If lifestyle changes are not enough and the symptoms of menopause continue and are difficult to tolerate, there are medications that can be very effective in managing postmenopausal symptoms without increasing your risk of breast cancer. Talk to your doctor about strategies that will alleviate your symptoms without increasing your breast cancer risk.

We do things every day—driving in a car, crossing the street, flying in airplanes—that involve minimal risk; we weigh the pros and cons and make the right decision for ourselves. Similarly, there are women who choose to take HRT knowing that there is an increased risk for breast cancer. For many, it's a lifestyle choice. For women who are not at an increased risk of breast cancer and who have difficult symptoms of menopause, it can be reasonable to take HRT for three to five years to get through the most difficult symptoms.

For example, one of our colleagues had such difficulty sleeping when she became menopausal that it was affecting her ability to concentrate. She tried for several months to manage her symptoms naturally, but ultimately chose to go on HRT; she felt much better as a result. Many years later, she was found to have atypical cells in one of her breasts and stopped the hormone treatment. Afterward, she didn't experience the symptoms that she had during those first few years of menopause and didn't regret that she had taken HRT. It's not uncommon that women who need HRT require a two-to-three-year course to get through the most difficult times of menopause and can stop after this time period with no further symptoms.

Arm yourself with the information about HRT and increased risk of breast cancer, and make the best decision for you. We hope you choose to never start HRT if you already have an increased risk for breast cancer, but the choice is yours, of course. This book is about empowering women with the information they need to make the best decision for them.

Most breast cancers in postmenopausal women are estrogen- and progesterone-receptor positive. That means that these cancers are fueled by the hormone estrogen. Estrogen-receptor-positive (ER-positive) cancers are often less aggressive than breast cancers that don't have these receptors. When ER-positive cancers are diagnosed early, they may be treated with antiestrogen drugs, such as tamoxifen and aromatase inhibitors. Chemotherapy may not be needed. If diagnosed later when there is lymph node involvement, even hormone-receptor-positive cancers likely require chemotherapy.

Hormonal therapy—which isn't the same as hormone replacement therapy but rather a treatment for cancers that are driven by estrogen—works by lowering the amount of estrogen in the body or by blocking the action of estrogen on breast cancer cells. There's an enzyme that can convert natural androgens in our body to estrogen, even when women are postmenopausal, called aromatase. Aromatase inhibitors stop the production of estrogen, thereby halting the availability of estrogen to the breast cancer cells. Aromatase inhibitors include Arimidex (anastrozole), Aromasin (exemestane), and Femara (letrozole). Aromatase inhibitors have been shown to be more effective at reducing breast cancer recurrence in postmenopausal women and are now used more often than tamoxifen to treat women who've gone through menopause.

Tamoxifen, a selective estrogen receptor modulator (SERM), is one of the most well-known hormonal therapies used. Tamoxifen prevents the estrogen receptors on breast cancer cells from connecting to estrogen, which they need to divide and grow. It acts like an antiestrogen in breast cells and an estrogen in tissues like the uterus and the bones. This is good, since SERMs can strengthen the bones and delay osteoporosis (bone thinning). Tamoxifen can be used to treat both premenopausal and postmenopausal women. It's used most often for premenopausal women, but also for postmenopausal women with osteoporosis.

For many years, the standard of care was for a woman to take hormonal therapy for five years for the treatment of breast cancer. In 2012 and 2013, large studies found that ten years of tamoxifen lowered breast cancer recurrence, reduced the number of breast cancer deaths, and improved overall survival. For women who already have osteoporosis, tamoxifen may be recommended over an aromatase inhibitor to help with bone issues as well.

While taking tamoxifen for ten years instead of five offers benefits and is generally the current recommendation, it does have side effects, some of them serious. Hot flashes and night sweats are common tamoxifen side effects. In rare cases, tamoxifen can cause blood clots, and it may increase the risk of endometrial cancer. The benefits of taking tamoxifen for ten years have to be weighed against the side effects. This is something you should discuss with your doctor.

Some research suggests that taking Femara, an aromatase inhibitor, for ten years instead of five may benefit women who have tolerated the first five years of therapy well, but currently, the data isn't conclusive. Taking an aromatase inhibitor for ten years isn't the standard of care, but most medical oncologists will assess symptoms at five to seven years to determine if an aromatase inhibitor should be continued. Like all drugs, aromatase inhibitors have side effects. The most common is joint pain. These drugs can also cause heart problems and decreased bone mass (osteopenia, osteoporosis).

CHEMOTHERAPY AND ER-POSITIVE BREAST CANCER

When it comes to other aspects of treatment for early ER-positive breast cancer, you may be wondering, "If I'm being treated with hormonal therapy, won't I get additional benefit from adding chemotherapy?"

Not necessarily. This is where we're truly moving into personalized medicine. There are now tests that take a woman's tumor sample, removed at the time of biopsy or surgery, and test it for the expression of twenty-one genes: sixteen cancer-related genes and five reference genes. Two of these tests are Oncotype DX and MammaPrint (see page 47 for more about these). The result is a recurrence score where a woman's tumor biology determines whether chemotherapy will be beneficial for her individually. Women with a low recurrence score do not benefit from additional chemotherapy; women who have a high recurrence score do. This personalized information is useful when a woman has ER-positive breast cancer. In our practice, the surgeon orders the test so that the information is available for the medical oncologist when they first meet with you in order to make the best recommendations. If you have ER-positive breast cancer, be certain to ask one of your doctors, likely your surgeon, to send your tumor for this test.

When Christy and Rachel began caring for women with breast cancer, all women with a breast cancer that was half an inch or larger were recommended to undergo chemotherapy, since we didn't have any way to determine who would benefit from chemotherapy and who would not. Today, we do—which is really quite incredible. Now only those women who will benefit from chemotherapy receive it. Treatment is based on tumor biology, even if the tumor is large.

The next question is, could women with more advanced HR-positive breast cancer with lymph node involvement be spared chemotherapy if they had low recurrence scores? Surprisingly enough, the answer is different for postmenopausal than premenopausal women. Postmenopausal women with this particular type of breast cancer didn't benefit from chemotherapy, but premenopausal women did. Many postmenopausal women may now be able to safely skip chemotherapy based on these advances in personalized genomic medicine.[7]

BREAST CONSERVATION AND PROSTHESIS

For postmenopausal women diagnosed with breast cancer that's contained in a small part of the breast, most breast surgeons recommend breast conservation (also known as lumpectomy or partial mastectomy), where only the tumor and a small margin of normal surrounding tissue are removed. A standard mastectomy removes the entire breast. For women with large tumors or more than one tumor in different parts of the breast, a mastectomy may be the only option. Postmenopausal women who need a mastectomy are generally candidates for reconstruction and can generally expect excellent cosmetic results. For those who want to keep their breasts, particularly if they have larger breasts, there's the option of having an oncoplastic reduction as part of their treatment, where a plastic surgeon performs a breast reduction while the cancerous tissue is being removed and a lift on the other breast so the two are the same size.

A lumpectomy or partial mastectomy is almost always accompanied by radiation; studies have clearly demonstrated that without radiation, the risk of the cancer recurring after a lumpectomy is increased. Research is underway to evaluate whether women over seventy with a low risk of recurrence can forgo radiation therapy, but we don't have conclusive results yet. In many cases, the answer is no, but for some women, it may be possible; this is something you should discuss with your doctor.

Both lumpectomy with radiation and mastectomy achieve equal survival results. However, every woman facing the difficult decision of choosing between a mastectomy and a lumpectomy must have a clear picture of the choices and their consequences.

It's important to have realistic expectations about what is possible after a lumpectomy or breast conservation. With the skill of a competent surgeon, the cosmetic results are generally very good. But if a portion of a woman's breast is removed, it can't possibly look exactly the same as the other breast. Often after radiation therapy, there are other physical changes such as redness and tenderness or even fat necrosis, lumps caused by the body's healing process.

The most frequent cosmetic consequence following a lumpectomy is that the breasts are asymmetric or changed in shape. If there's a significant difference in the size or shape of your breasts after a lumpectomy, a plastic surgeon can improve the appearance of the treated breast by making it larger to match the native breast, whether with a small implant or by moving fat from other parts of the body to increase the size of the surgically treated breast (this is called fat grafting). Alternatively, the plastic surgeon can reduce the size of the native breast to make it more closely match the breast that was treated for cancer. There are many approaches to increase the symmetry of your breasts during the initial treatment of breast cancer or after. That's why it's important to have an extensive discussion with your plastic surgeon about what you would like, what's possible, and what types of surgery or procedures will most closely achieve the desired result. Remember, it's very important that you seek out a plastic surgeon with extensive experience in breast reconstruction. Don't hesitate to ask how often they do these types of procedures and what percentage of their practice is devoted to breast surgery. These are very important questions, as both experience and expertise are critical to achieving the best outcome. Insurance should cover any of these procedures.

Although many of us who are postmenopausal care how we look as we age, many of our physical features change and we learn to live with increasing imperfection. Many postmenopausal women come to feel this way about their postlumpectomy changes. Women are most often satisfied with the cosmetic outcome of their lumpectomy, even if there's a significant difference in the appearance of their breasts. The imbalances and imperfections are rarely so bad that they're noticeable when you're fully dressed.

For women who are not interested in having plastic surgery,

there are prostheses called breast equalizers. These silicone breast forms can be placed inside a special bra that holds them in place in order to make your treated breast appear the same size as your native breast under your clothes. Most insurance plans cover the cost of breast equalizers and whole-breast prosthetics for women who undergo mastectomy without reconstruction.

For Christy's mother, breast conservation was the obvious choice in 1997 when she was diagnosed with her first cancer at the age of sixty. None of the family knew their family history of breast cancer at the time. Oddly enough, the prevailing trend in genetic testing in those days was to not test women age sixty or older for genetic risk of breast cancer. Christy's mother had no idea whether she was BRCA positive or not.

Her breasts were small, but the cancerous tumor was also small, so that was an advantage. She had surgery with one of the excellent surgeons Christy had trained with at Memorial Sloan Kettering Cancer Center. The final pathology showed a small one-centimeter tumor with clear margins and negative sentinel lymph nodes. Having cancer was scary, but her prognosis was excellent. If she had had surgery one year prior, she would have needed an axillary lymph node dissection, but thanks to science, she was offered the less-invasive sentinel lymph node biopsy procedure rather than the full axillary lymph node dissection.

Because her tumor was ER-positive, Christy's mother was treated with tamoxifen. No chemotherapy was indicated. Back then, there were no tests such as Oncotype DX to determine tumor biology, so treatment was based on the size of the tumor and whether it had spread to the lymph nodes. The entire process for her first bout of cancer was relatively easy. If her tumor had been larger, she would have needed a mastectomy. If it had spread to one of her lymph nodes, she would have needed chemotherapy. If she had been more particular about her breasts, she might have opted for more surgeries to even them out, but she never did. No one could tell she'd had surgery for breast cancer. She was beautiful before her breast cancer and she was just as beautiful afterward. Her recovery was quick, and she was working in her garden soon after the surgery. She was able to go about her normal activities during radiation and had no side effects from the treatment.

VARIABLES

Family history, genetic mutations, large breasts, age, and a wide range of health issues are just a few of the considerations facing postmenopausal women dealing with breast cancer. There are so many variables in breast cancer treatment (for women at any stage of life), and with so many choices to make, our patients often feel ill-equipped to make the best decision. If you're feeling that way, rest assured that many other women in your position feel the same way, too.

Family History

A significant number of postmenopausal women in our practice have a family history of breast cancer. As a result, many of our patients want to minimize their chances of ever having to deal with breast cancer again. Choosing mastectomies in both breasts can essentially remove the possibility of developing cancer in the opposite breast.

Brook Jensen was diagnosed with early-stage breast cancer at the age of fifty-four. She had gone through menopause at the age of fifty-one. She had successful breast conservation surgery with a partial mastectomy and sentinel lymph node biopsy. She didn't know at the time that she had a family history of breast cancer. When she started discussing her diagnosis with her extended family, she learned of several other relatives who had also had breast cancer.

Brook underwent breast cancer treatment and was doing well, but ultimately chose to minimize her future risk with bilateral mastectomies and chose to not have any reconstruction, i.e., she went "flat." She said her breasts were not important to her or her husband, and she wanted to get back to work and her normal activities as quickly as possible. Brook avoided the process of reconstruction and has never regretted her decision. Within three weeks, she was back to working full time, and by four weeks, she was back to her regular exercise routine.

Three of Katie Tamarind's four sisters were diagnosed with postmenopausal breast cancer by the time we saw her. When Katie was diagnosed with a very early noninvasive breast cancer called ductal carcinoma in situ (DCIS) in her right breast at the age of fifty-six, she assumed that her family had a BRCA mutation. To her surprise, genetic testing showed that they didn't. But even though she was a candidate for breast conservation, she still decided to have bilateral preventive mastectomies. She was convinced her family history put her at an increased risk for breast cancer and wanted to reduce that risk at all costs. Katie's family history strongly suggests that there's a genetic component behind their cancers, and she may have a gene mutation that has not yet been identified. (Another, less likely possibility is environmental toxins. Katie and her sisters may have lived in an area with toxic conditions that they were unaware of that caused so many members of the same family to get cancer.)

Ultimately, Katie chose to have reconstruction using her own abdominal tissue. She loved the idea! Not only was she changing the family narrative of breast cancer, she was getting a tummy tuck, too. Now Katie has beautiful reconstructed breasts and a flat stomach. Katie is convinced this was the best choice for her, and was grateful she didn't need radiation or tamoxifen.

The number of genes known to be associated with an increased risk of breast cancer is constantly increasing. The availability of large data sets and centralized databases now allow for the more efficient and effective identification of genes associated with cancer at a faster rate than ever before. We're constantly gaining new information and insights into the causes and risks of cancer.

Genetics

We can now change the narrative of our family histories with cancer through genetic testing, proactive choices, and careful surveillance that can usually detect breast cancer in its earliest stages.

Two percent of women with Ashkenazi Jewish heritage have a genetic mutation for BRCA, which can be passed to them equally from their mothers or their fathers. In the general population, one in four hundred women overall have a BRCA gene; in Ashkenazi Jewish women, the risk is ten times higher, with one in forty having a gene. The incidence of deleterious genes associated with increased risk of cancer is higher in the Black community as well, although not as high as it is in the Ashkenazi Jewish population.

Ruth Somers already knew that her aunt had had breast cancer when she was postmenopausal. When Ruth was diagnosed with breast cancer at fifty-eight, she tested positive for a BRCA2 mutation. She knew that every cell in her body, not just the ones that had developed into cancer, had this same mutation. Having the mutation led to her decision to have preventive mastectomies, an obvious choice for her.

After speaking with one of our plastic surgeons to discuss reconstruction options, Ruth chose to have nipple-sparing mastectomies with implants. She was grateful she didn't need chemotherapy and was able to be treated with surgery and a daily aromatase inhibitor.

As a result of Ruth finding out about her own BRCA2 mutation, several of her daughters and nieces are going to be tested as well. This may be a positive consequence of breast cancer, but it's a difficult one. It's important to share information with your family that could help them make lifesaving decisions with awareness, and early intervention is critically important. Ruth shared with us that if any of her daughters test positive for the same mutation, they will likely choose to have preventive mastectomies themselves.

Large Breasts

For patients who have large breasts, there may be additional considerations. Delores Jenkins's breasts were so large that they caused pain in her shoulders and back. When she was diagnosed with breast cancer at the age of sixty-six and was advised to have a right mastectomy due to the extent of disease, she chose to also have a left mastectomy for cosmetic and, more important for her, comfort reasons. She didn't want to wear a prosthesis that would match her remaining breast. We offered her the option of having the left breast reduced so that it could be more easily matched with a prosthesis on the right, but she had no interest in keeping that breast. After her bilateral mastectomies, the pathology of the left breast, which was thought to be normal on preoperative imaging, showed breast cancer as well. She felt fortunate that she didn't have to endure additional future breast cancer treatments. Although this scenario—that is, that an incidental cancer is found in what was thought to be the healthy breast—is uncommon, it's certainly not unheard of. Invariably this further justifies the decision to undergo bilateral mastectomies.

Delores felt exceptionally empowered by her decision. When she made the choice not to have reconstruction, Christy gave her a prescription for mastectomy bras with prosthetics, but she never ordered them. The next time Dolores came for a follow-up visit, she laughed and said, "For the first time since I was eleven years old, I can go without a bra. I feel free!"

It's not uncommon for women to ultimately find a silver lining to the gray cloud of breast cancer. In Delores's case, it was the ability to go braless and be comfortable for the first time since she was a child.

For women who don't need or opt for a mastectomy but have large breasts, breast reduction can be an excellent option, even if their tumor is small, because it improves results from radiation. This is called an oncoplastic reduction mammoplasty and is discussed in more detail in chapter 9. The side effects from radiation, which can include skin irritation and redness and lymphedema (swelling that may require physical therapy treatment), can be greater for women with large breasts. Having the oncoplastic reduction before radiation therapy may minimize the side effects of radiation.

Age

In healthy young women, breast cancer surgery is low risk. For most patients, breast conservation is performed as an outpatient procedure. But as time goes on, age makes things more complicated for postmenopausal women. A woman who seemed young and vigorous after menopause at fifty-six may well be frailer when she's in her eighties. By that time, she may have other medical conditions that increase the risks associated with surgery. These issues need to be considered when making the difficult decisions a breast cancer diagnosis necessitates.

A *JAMA Surgery* study conducted at the University of California San Francisco followed almost six thousand nursing home residents for ten years after breast cancer surgery. Their average

age was eighty-two. Many had high rates of arthritis, diabetes, heart failure, and stroke. More than half suffered from cognitive impairment and needed help with everyday tasks.[8] These issues need to be considered when making decisions about breast cancer surgery, treatment, and reconstruction.

Unless there are imminent, life-threatening conditions at play, most women are treated with the same standard of care, regardless of age. It was thought that very old women diagnosed with breast cancer might be treated with less aggressive therapy, since there was a greater chance that they would die of other causes. However, that was not the case. In fact, when older women are not treated with the standard of care, they often do die from breast cancer. Therefore, it's important not to dismiss treating older women with state-of-the-art care, if they're healthy enough to tolerate it.[9] Advanced age should not mean women receive less effective, less intensive treatment.

Some women in their eighties are traveling the world, enjoying their careers, delighting in their families, or writing books about their lives. Grandma Moses, the famous artist who began painting in earnest at the age of seventy-eight, painted well into her nineties. Older women should not be treated as patients who are going to die soon and have nothing to live for!

One of our patients, Andrea Bernstein, was a fun-loving independent eighty-year-old at the center of a large, loving family with many friends around her. She was close to her daughters and grandchildren. She couldn't wait to see her son, whom she hadn't seen in over a year due to the COVID-19 pandemic.

With a history of a left breast cancer that had been treated with a lumpectomy and radiation therapy, Andrea diligently came in for annual mammograms. One year, her mammogram showed new calcifications in the left breast and a concerning mass in the right breast. We biopsied both and found cancer on the right.

A needle biopsy found that the left breast had atypia, abnormal cells that require surgical excision to make certain the adjacent cells are not more abnormal and cancerous.

Less-than-optimal treatment was out of the question for Andrea. Chronologically she was eighty, but physiologically and emotionally she was decades younger. She was thrilled that breast conservation was an option on the right breast, and had the atypia on her left breast excised. She knew that we would likely recommend a mastectomy on the left if there were cancer cells seen on the final pathology since she had already been treated with radiation in that breast. Luckily, there was no cancer on the left. She was given the option of not having radiation on the right because her tumor was low risk, and started taking the aromatase inhibitor Femara (letrozole). Andrea was willing to have a mastectomy if necessary, but she preferred not to, and is thankful to have been able to keep both of her breasts. She continues with close screening and surveillance but is otherwise living her wonderful, full life.

Some recommendations for breast cancer screening suggest that women over seventy-four avoid screening altogether. It isn't because mammography is ineffective in older women. In fact, mammography is easier to interpret in older women since they tend to have less dense breast tissue, making it harder for cancers to hide as they can in women with dense breast tissue. It's not that the risk of breast cancer decreases with age—quite the opposite. The risk of cancer continues to increase throughout life. In fact, studies demonstrate that if you stop screening older women for breast cancer, they die of breast cancer more often. The reason some organizations don't recommend mammography for women over seventy-four is that most studies that evaluate the impact of screening mammography do not include women over that age. But just because those women weren't included in the studies doesn't mean it doesn't work. It does. Therefore, our recommendation, and the recommendation of many organizations and societies, is that women who have a five-year or greater life expectancy, regardless of age, continue to undergo annual screening mammography. Christy and Rachel have patients in their eighties and nineties who come every year for their mammograms and clinical examinations. The women are happy to be proactive, and treating them is an honor.

Health Issues

It's very common for postmenopausal women to have at least one other unrelated health issue at the time they're diagnosed with breast cancer. These preexisting conditions may be things as common as high blood pressure or high cholesterol, common medical issues that don't significantly impact breast cancer therapy decisions. In most cases, we're able to diagnose, treat, and operate to eliminate breast cancer with the intention of curing postmenopausal women, even when they're not in the peak of health. However, when women have significant life-threatening medical conditions, such as end-stage heart or kidney disease or significant cognitive decline, the preexisting condition may influence their treatment options. Many chemotherapeutic regimens need to be altered in patients whose hearts are significantly compromised by disease. Sometimes the decision is made to not undergo conventional therapy, such as chemotherapy or even surgery, due to coexisting severe health issues. This is, of course, rare. But these considerations must be included in the final therapeutic decisions. Depending on the woman's condition, chemotherapy, breast conservation therapy, or mastectomies may not be advisable.[10] However, most of the research on the effectiveness of cancer treatments is derived from clinical trials that exclude women over seventy who have breast cancer and other preexisting health issues.[11]

CHOOSING FOR YOURSELF

Mammography is an excellent examination and has been instrumental in the 40 percent decrease in deaths from breast cancer we've seen over the past two decades.[12] Inevitably, searching for and finding more cancers also means identifying more benign masses as well. At this point, the only way to tell if a breast mass is cancerous is by doing a biopsy. These days, all biopsies should be performed minimally invasively with a core needle rather than by surgical excision. If the mass is seen on a mammogram, the biopsy will done by mammographic guidance; if it's seen on ultrasound, it will be done by ultrasound guidance. Sometimes it's seen only on MRI, when an MRI biopsy is performed to confirm the presence of a cancer.

The good news is that most postmenopausal women are candidates for breast conservation, which is what we generally recommend. But for women who aren't interested in keeping their breasts, it isn't unreasonable to ask for a mastectomy or bilateral mastectomies. Again, there is no right decision about whether to do a mastectomy versus a partial mastectomy/lumpectomy with radiation therapy if you have the choice. Decisions regarding mastectomy with or without reconstruction are very personal. Rarely, but occasionally, surgery can be avoided altogether for women who have ER-positive tumors and are not candidates for surgery. Taking an aromatase inhibitor or tamoxifen will likely not only keep the tumor from growing but may even shrink it. These are difficult and often complicated choices for every woman who faces them. Your best solution is to be as well-informed as possible and confer with your doctor, your family, and your support system before making your decision. As we've discussed throughout this book, it's a very personal decision.

Common Questions to Discuss with Your Care Team

For pathology-related questions, please refer to the Common Questions list in chapter 3.

Am I a candidate for keeping my breast?

What's the difference between a lumpectomy and a partial mastectomy?

Do I need to have a sentinel lymph node biopsy?

If I keep my breast, will I need radiation? If so, do I need radiation to the entire breast or just the part of the breast where the cancer is located?

What are the side effects of radiation?

Is it possible that I'll need chemotherapy?

How will I feel, and what should I expect when I'm having chemotherapy?

What is hormonal therapy?

What are the side effects of the recommended hormonal therapy?

What if I have osteopenia or osteoporosis?

What are the chances that my cancer will come back?

Why do I need to have my breast removed? Is there an option to keep it even if cancer was detected in more than one area of the breast?

If I have a mastectomy, can I avoid chemotherapy?

If I have a mastectomy, will I need radiation?

If I need the cancerous breast removed, what should I do with the other breast?

Do I have the option of having both breasts removed even if I'm a candidate for keeping my breast if that's my preference?

Am I a candidate for reconstruction if I need a mastectomy?

What if I don't want reconstruction?

Will I go home after surgery? If not, how long will I be in the hospital?

Do I have the option of staying in the hospital overnight if that's my preference?

Will I need help at home after surgery?

What is my expected recovery, and can I do normal activities at home?

Will I need a drain?

Will I need physical therapy?

What about immunotherapy or clinical trials? Are any appropriate for me, and should I consider either of these options?

If I'm not interested in having surgery because of my age or medical issues, do I have the option of taking medication and avoiding surgery and radiation? If so, how will I be followed?

CHAPTER 8

Your Mastectomy Options

B reast cancer is one of the few diseases where you have many choices about what kind of surgery you'll undergo and which treatments you'll receive. What other tumors have surgeons asking patients how far they should go with the surgery?[1]

From 2002 to 2012, *three times* as many women with invasive cancer in one breast chose to have double mastectomies for prevention, even when a partial mastectomy in one breast was medically possible. In 2013, after her mother died of ovarian cancer and she tested positive for a BRCA1 mutation, Angelina Jolie made a very public decision about undergoing preventive mastectomies.[2] Although her public decision was an affirmation to many young women with BRCA mutations and other high-risk situations, the trend toward more prophylactic mastectomy started long before her decision.

Thanks to the astonishing advances in medicine over the past few decades, women at increased risk of or who've been diagnosed with breast cancer have more choices now than ever before. There are, of course, constraints as a result of your medical situation. But in many cases, you can choose to remove only the cancer, remove an entire breast with cancer, remove the other breast as a precaution, save the nipples (or not), reconstruct your breasts with your own tissue or implants, or not have reconstruction done at all. One thing is certain: there's an increasing trend toward performing preventive mastectomies for women at increased risk as well as to remove the other breast to avoid the possibility of future cancer in women with a breast cancer diagnosis.

Increasingly, women with breast cancer are opting for larger surgeries to reduce their risk of facing cancer again in the future. A partial mastectomy, the most common procedure to treat breast cancer, takes about an hour, and the patient can often go home that day, although they will likely have to return for radiation treatment. The cosmetic results are usually excellent, even if the breasts are no longer symmetric. When done for small tumors, there may be no difference in the appearance of the breasts. When a single mastectomy is performed, reconstruction is offered, but the reconstructed breast may not perfectly match the remaining breast, and hospital admission is generally required. A double mastectomy with reconstruction takes at least four hours, with a longer recovery time, and generally requires other surgeries to address the consequences of the first.[3] In the United States today, 65 percent of women with newly diagnosed breast cancer choose partial mastectomies and 35 percent choose full mastectomies.[4] For now, that seems to be an American trend. Women in Berlin and Seoul are four times more likely to choose partial mastectomies.[5] Considerations are based not only on medical factors but on social and psychological factors as well.

Even in the United States, undergoing mastectomy for breast cancer where partial mastectomy or lumpectomy is a viable option is controversial. There are surgeons who have been outspoken critics of the rising trend in preventive mastectomies. Some studies have shown that patients overestimate the risk of getting cancer in the opposite breast, and that those with a risk of 5 percent or less should be discouraged from undergoing mastectomy. If the risk is 10 percent, 15 percent, or 30 percent, the decision should be tailored to each patient and weighed against their personal risk of incurring metastatic cancer at a distant location in the body.[6]

However, it's very important to remember that many of the people making these recommendations haven't walked in the shoes of the women who need to make these decisions and live with the consequences. As a breast cancer survivor, Rachel has difficulty with some recommendations of surgeons who undoubtedly have their patients' best interests in mind but who clearly have no idea what it's like to be reminded that you're a cancer patient every time you look in the mirror and see the asymmetry of your breasts, or deal with the daily concern of cancer recurrence. It's for this and so many other reasons that we chose to share our expertise, experience, and personal decisions with you in this book. When we recommend options to our patients, they know we've experienced similar situations and have used our professional expertise and personal experience. Remember, when you're making these critical decisions, well-meaning and expert physicians usually haven't shared your experiences as we have, and when they offer recommendations, it's without the insight that comes from being in a similar situation.

A partial mastectomy is indeed less invasive, and offers women the hope of a long, fulfilling life when they're no longer "cancer patients." For most women, a lumpectomy or partial mastectomy with a quicker recovery that results in keeping their breasts is the right decision. The doctors you consult may have completely different reactions than you would have to the same situation. That's fine. It's human nature. Never forget that you're the one who must live with the results. When you're considering your options, it doesn't matter what your doctors would be comfortable with. Ask yourself what *you* will be most comfortable with.

Since the choice you make will impact the way you look and feel for the rest of your life, it's essential that you know all the facts and implications before you decide. You need time to think over the options carefully and ask yourself questions you may have never considered before: If you remove the cancer in one breast, how much will you worry about getting cancer in the other one? Which do you find more unsettling: getting scans every six months with the possibility of biopsies to make sure you don't have cancer, or potentially having several surgeries for breast reconstruction? If members of your family have had breast cancer, would you choose the uncertainty of not knowing whether you'll get breast cancer, or eliminate the possibility once and for all?

The fundamental difference between preventive mastectomies and careful surveillance is the difference between certainty and hope. Preventive mastectomies ensure that you most likely will never get breast cancer. Surveillance—including regular scans and potential biopsies—rely on the assumption that if a cancer is found, it will be found early.

WHAT IS A MASTECTOMY?

- **Partial mastectomy.** The removal of a cancerous tumor and some normal breast tissue around the tumor. It's also known as lumpectomy, breast conservation, or excisional biopsy, but most breast surgeons now refer to this procedure as a partial mastectomy.
- **Simple mastectomy.** The removal of the entire breast but not the muscle under the breast. There are three variations:
- *Modified radical mastectomy:* A simple mastectomy with removal of the axillary lymph nodes because cancer has spread to the nodes.
- *Nipple-sparing mastectomy:* A simple mastectomy that saves

the nipple and areola. A sentinel lymph node biopsy will also be done if cancer is present.

- *Skin-sparing mastectomy:* A simple mastectomy that saves the skin of the breast to provide an envelope for breast reconstruction. This can be done with and without nipple sparing. A sentinel lymph node biopsy will also be done if cancer is present.
- **Radical mastectomy.** The removal of the entire breast, chest wall muscles, and lymph nodes. This option is more historical and is rarely done today. It's only necessary if the cancer has grown into the chest muscle.

As we discuss in chapter 9, breast reconstruction has dramatically improved in recent years. Many women choose to reduce or enlarge the size of their original breasts and are pleased with the results. Nipple-sparing mastectomies are a popular option for cosmetic reasons, as long as the tissue behind the nipple and areola is cancer-free. All mastectomies result in permanent numbness of the breast. Nipple sensation is lost, and breastfeeding isn't possible since the mammary glands have been removed. If tissue to be used for reconstruction has been taken from another area of the body (such as the thigh, abdomen, or buttocks), that area may not regain feeling, either. Plastic surgeons are exploring the option of doing nerve reconstructions to help maintain some nipple sensation (this will be discussed in chapter 11).

That said, almost half (46 percent) of all women choose *not* to do reconstruction after a mastectomy.[7] Some are not candidates for medical reasons. For example, surgeons will recommend against reconstruction for women whose cancer has spread to their skin or who have many medical issues that make a shorter surgery the safer option. Others prefer to recover more quickly and avoid the more complicated surgeries involved with reconstruction. Many prefer to go flat and are satisfied with that option, particularly if they feel supported by their surgeon and family.[8]

Simple Mastectomy

When a simple mastectomy is performed without reconstruction, the breast tissue, nipple, areola, and extra skin of the breast are all removed. The final appearance is a flat chest with a straight horizontal incision where the breast was. It's not uncommon for there to be some extra skin or fat on the sides or in the middle, which we refer to as "dog ears." These can be bothersome to patients cosmetically and can cause discomfort when wearing a bra with a prosthesis. A rather uncomplicated, same-day surgical procedure performed by your breast surgeon or plastic surgeon can usually correct this.

Although the cosmetic result is much better when reconstruction is performed at the time of the mastectomy, it's always possible to do reconstruction later. In some cases, women may need to have the cancerous tissue removed right away, but the demands of their lives make it difficult to do a series of reconstructive surgeries. Others must wait to schedule reconstruction at a later date when their breast cancer is under better control and they have completed all treatments.

One of our patients, Kathy Daniels, was diagnosed with advanced breast cancer in 2001. We were concerned about doing immediate reconstruction due to the extent of disease, so she had a modified radical mastectomy without reconstruction. She was treated with chemotherapy and radiation. After all her treatment was complete, she decided to undergo reconstruction using her own tissue (latissimus flap) and an implant. While the time having a flat chest was difficult for her, she was extremely pleased with her final reconstructed breast—it looked nothing like her normal breast, but in clothing it matched her unaffected breast well.

Your reconstructed breasts won't be like your previous breasts. It's part of the new normal that any woman with breast cancer or who undergoes mastectomies must embrace. As we will discuss in chapter 9, reconstructed breasts can be beautiful. In fact, they can be perkier and have a better shape than your native breast, especially if you've breastfed a child.

For some women, the decision is about recovery. The recovery from a simple mastectomy is much easier and faster than recovery when reconstruction is done, and there's usually little pain.

Christy's mother is a good example. With her first cancer in 1997, she opted for breast conservation and had a sentinel lymph node biopsy (a cutting-edge procedure at the time), thus avoiding a complete axillary lymph node dissection. This meant she had the first draining lymph node from the breast removed, rather than all of them, which was then the standard procedure. It reduced her risk of having lymphedema or swelling of the arm down to 2 or 3 percent from around 25 percent. She breezed through radiation and tamoxifen, from which she had no side effects, and had decent cosmetic results. She was cancer-free for thirteen years.

When she was diagnosed with cancer in the other breast thirteen years later, the decision to have bilateral mastectomies was straightforward for her. The cancer didn't show up on a mammogram or ultrasound and involved many lymph nodes, which meant she was going to require both chemotherapy and radiation. She didn't want to bother trying to match the other breast with a prosthesis and was not interested in having reconstruction. In addition, she wanted the quickest and easiest recovery possible, particularly since there was a planned family reunion cruise a month later, which she was committed to being part of. She underwent

the surgery and was able to go on the cruise, then started chemotherapy shortly after her return. This is an example of how other
plans can impact your decision to have or forgo reconstruction.

Age also often plays a role in the decision. Marlene Young
found a mass in her right breast at the age of thirty-eight and
was diagnosed with cancer in several areas of her breast. As a
result of the multiple cancers, a mastectomy, either nipple sparing
or skin sparing, was the only possible surgical option. Initially,
Marlene was treated with chemotherapy because the tumor was
triple-negative. She had an excellent response to chemotherapy,
and while she had the option of reconstruction, she chose against
it because she was busy with her career, and as a single mother,
and she wanted an easier and faster recovery. She chose to forgo
reconstruction due to the potential that it would require several
surgeries. She chose to have both breasts removed not only for
symmetry but also because she never wanted to go through chemotherapy again. She knew that reconstruction was an option in
the future, but was not interested at that moment.

Another patient, Karen Hughes, was treated for breast cancer
at the age of fifty-four with a partial mastectomy and sentinel
lymph node biopsy followed by radiation. At the time of her
diagnosis, she considered having mastectomies, but wanted the
easiest surgery possible because her job was stressful and she
could not take much time off. About two years after her surgery,
she was found to have atypical hyperplasia in the other breast.
Rather than the recommended surgical excision to exclude the
possibility of cancer in that region of the breast, she decided to
have bilateral mastectomies without reconstruction. Things had
calmed down at work, so it was a good time to do the surgery,
and she and her husband both agreed that it was the best decision for her. She was not interested in having reconstruction and
looked forward to going from relatively large breasts to being

flat. She felt empowered to not only never have to have another mammogram but also to never have to wear a bra again.

There are so many options for reconstruction, as well as the option to forgo reconstruction completely. No single decision is right for every woman—these monumental decisions are based on your own medical situation, needs, and wants. These women made different choices based on their circumstances, their risk tolerance, and their personal preference. There are so many considerations and so many "right" decisions.

Nipple-Sparing Mastectomy

A nipple-sparing mastectomy involves removal of the breast tissue behind the skin of the breast and the nipple and areolar complex, leaving them intact. It can only be done if reconstruction is planned. Keeping the woman's own skin and nipples results in a more natural-appearing breast after reconstruction.

If a patient is a good candidate for the procedure, the cosmetic result is usually better than a skin-sparing mastectomy, where the nipple is removed at the time of surgery. The incision for nipple- and skin-sparing mastectomies can be in the fold under the breast, so after this procedure, there may be no visible scars. This is an excellent option for many women, but especially for young women. They won't have to explain their situation every time they're in a locker room or in a dressing room shopping with their friends.

Some women are not candidates for a nipple-sparing mastectomy because their breasts are too large. If they prefer the option of having a nipple-sparing mastectomy, the plastic surgeon can often perform a staging reduction mammoplasty to get the nipple and areola where they need to be. Both breasts first are reduced so that they're symmetric, and the nipple-sparing mastectomy with reconstruction can then be performed eight to twelve weeks later.

We did this option for Jennifer Canter. She had a known BRCA2 mutation and decided it was time to have mastectomies. Her breasts were large, so she was not a candidate for nipple-sparing mastectomies, but keeping her nipples was important to her. She met with our plastic surgeon, who agreed that having reduction mammoplasties first would enable her to keep her nipples and improve her cosmetic results. She had the reduction surgery, which required about two weeks off from work. While she knew that she could have the mastectomy surgery three months later, she waited six months because the timing was better for her. She had the nipple-sparing mastectomies with implant reconstructions right after Thanksgiving and took advantage of things being quiet over the holidays to recover.

There are many different incisions used in surgery. One incision is made under the fold of the breast: the inframammary fold. Other incisions are more lateral, where they begin near the edge of the areola and extend toward the outer portion of the breast. For patients who had a staging reduction mammoplasty like Jennifer, the prior vertical incisions that extend from the edge of the areola to the bottom of the breast and then along the inframammary fold are used.

In these cases, all visible breast tissue is removed. In the past, this was called a subcutaneous mastectomy, but with that kind of mastectomy, tissue behind the nipple and areola were left behind. A nipple-sparing mastectomy is different because no matter what incision is used, tissue beneath the nipple and areola is removed and checked for cancer. If cancer is detected, the nipple and areola are removed, converting the procedure into a skin-sparing mastectomy.

When Christy had her own preventive mastectomies, she was an excellent candidate for a nipple-sparing procedure because her breasts were not large and the nipples were in the correct position. She doesn't have much body fat, so implants were the best reconstructive option. Christy chose her colleague Anita McSwain, who did her mother's mastectomies, to also do hers. Anita hadn't done nipple-sparing mastectomies before because the procedure was relatively new, so Christy worked with her in the operating room to show her the technique. When it was time for Christy's surgery, she was confident that Anita was ready, and she did an amazing job.

When Christy's mother was making decisions about her own mastectomies, she told Christy it didn't bother her to remove her breasts since she was not particularly attached to them. They were small and not symmetric due to her prior cancer surgery on the left breast. Christy wasn't attached to hers, either, since they had always been small and were even smaller after breastfeeding three children. Unlike her mother, Christy liked the idea of doing reconstruction, and finally was able to have larger breasts that fit her body. The numbness doesn't bother her, and she continues to be delighted with the results.

Skin-Sparing Mastectomy

A skin-sparing simple mastectomy saves most of the breast's skin for reconstruction but removes the nipple and areola. This is the best option for women who are interested in having reconstruction but either are not good candidates for nipple-sparing due to location of the cancer or size of the breast, or have no interest in keeping the nipple. As with a simple mastectomy, a sentinel lymph node biopsy is performed if there's a known cancer. This type of mastectomy is still possible if cancer is found in the nodes, requiring an axillary lymph node dissection.

In our discussion of reconstruction in chapter 9, you'll find more details about the time required for the procedure, hospital stay, and recovery. For women who have skin-sparing mastectomies, a nipple and areola can be re-created by the plastic surgeon several months after the surgery. As with all mastectomies, neither the skin nor the nipple retains any sensation.

When Rachel decided to have preventive mastectomies in 1996, nipple-sparing mastectomies were not an option; so much has changed since then. The BRCA mutation had only been identified several years earlier. Widespread genetic testing was not yet available, but Rachel had access to early testing and found, as she suspected, that she was a BRCA1 mutation carrier. Although she had suspected that she might be a carrier of the genetic mutation, definitively learning that she had the mutation resulted in her being proactive. She scheduled bilateral preventive mastectomies with transverse rectus abdominis myocutaneous (TRAM) flap reconstructions (see chapter 9), which use abdominal fat to re-create the breasts. Rachel chose this reconstruction because she preferred to do a procedure that would not require additional surgery in the future. Implants don't last forever, and since she was only thirty-seven years old, it was highly likely that if she chose implants, they would need to be replaced several times in the future. Because Rachel has frequently gained and lost weight throughout her life, it was comforting to know that with this choice, her breasts would change as her weight did. Although the surgery was longer and the recovery more difficult, this choice was the right one for Rachel, and she was comfortable making it.

Between scheduling her prophylactic mastectomies and her surgical date, Rachel found her own cancer while trying some new ultrasound equipment. Since she had a cancer in her left breast, she needed to have a full axillary lymph node dissection as well. Although Rachel was offered sentinel lymph node biopsy, it was truly in its infancy at the time, and there was little long-term data about the impact of this procedure. As a result of the lymph node removal, Rachel is careful with her left arm, avoiding cuts or injections in that arm to prevent lymphedema (swelling).

One of our patients, Cara Henry, elected to have bilateral mastectomies at the age of thirty-six because of her BRCA1 mutation. She had other medical issues and was concerned that if she were later diagnosed with breast cancer, she would have a difficult time if chemotherapy was necessary. While she liked the idea of keeping her nipples, she was not a candidate because her breasts were too large and her nipples were not in the correct locations to be spared. She wanted to have the fewest surgeries possible and therefore chose to have skin-sparing mastectomies with immediate implant reconstructions. She was able to have these procedures in one surgery and therefore had only one recovery. She's happy with her results, and thankful to not require any other surgeries, and more important, she doesn't need to worry about a diagnosis of breast cancer or the possibility that she will have to undergo chemotherapy.

MASTECTOMY DOES NOT IMPROVE SURVIVAL

As you make your own choice, it's important to realize that there's almost no difference in survival or recurrence rates between partial mastectomy with radiation and mastectomy for women diagnosed with breast cancer. This is surprising to many women, and it's not uncommon when they're first diagnosed to want the breast removed, hoping that it will mean no other treatment will be necessary. The risk of local recurrence after a mastectomy is 1 to 3 percent.[9] The risk of a local recurrence after a partial mastectomy is 5 to 8 percent.[10] If a recurrence does occur, the survival rate is the same as if a mastectomy had been performed at the time of the initial surgery. Having a mastectomy may eliminate the need for radiation, but other treatments will likely be necessary.

When we say that mastectomies don't improve your survival rate, we mean that in a very specific way. If the cancer is removed with breast conservation surgery and then the remaining cancer cells are killed with radiation, the cancer may be completely gone. Even if that original cancer returns, having a mastectomy to treat the original cancer doesn't change survival outcomes. Removing the entire breast at the time of initial diagnosis doesn't improve the situation. However, studies looking at a woman's survival from an initial cancer do not look at her survival from subsequent cancers. Removing the breasts essentially eliminates the possibility of getting another cancer but doesn't change your survival rate from the original cancer.

For most patients, the risk of getting a new cancer is small and shouldn't be the only reason to choose a mastectomy. Many surgeons are adamant that patients should choose partial mastectomy if they're candidates for it. As long as they don't have a genetic mutation that raises their risk of a new cancer, many physicians feel they should discourage their patients from having mastectomies. In fact, surgeons are expected to advise patients who are candidates for breast conservation against the option of mastectomies. We don't share this opinion. We believe that our responsibility as physicians is to inform our patients fully, and then let them make their own decisions. We aren't here to judge. Since we've been through this decision-making process in our own lives—for ourselves and our loved ones—we're poignantly aware of how many factors weigh into these critical decisions. Every woman's decision is based on different issues. It's essential that you know the facts, but the decision you ultimately make is personal. And we, as physicians, are here to support and respect your decision.

It's heartbreaking to treat patients whose surgeon strongly recommended breast conservation or a mastectomy on one breast (a unilateral mastectomy) who then later get cancer in the other breast and generally choose to have a contralateral mastectomy. It's devastating emotionally for them to realize that they could have avoided a second cancer by doing a preventive mastectomy, particularly if chemotherapy is necessary. Some have died as a result of their second cancer. Christy's mother was one of them; she would not have died from her first cancer. Of course, this is not the case with the overwhelming majority of women who undergo partial mastectomy. Most do just fine.

For those with the BRCA mutations, there is now data showing that mastectomies can impact survival whether they're done before[11] or after a diagnosis of cancer.[12]

INSURANCE COVERAGE

Many women ask whether insurance will cover having a contralateral mastectomy when a mastectomy is necessary for cancer, or bilateral mastectomies even if they're candidates for breast conservation. Most insurance companies will cover the procedures, and are required by law to cover reconstruction or mastectomy bras and prosthetics for those who elect not to undergo reconstruction. Most insurance will also cover preventive mastectomies for women who are at an increased risk due to a genetic mutation, family history, or other factor as was discussed in chapter 5. Insurance will also cover mastectomies for women who first undergo breast-conservation surgery but then change their minds and elect to proceed with mastectomies at a later date, as long as the woman's physician agrees. Being comfortable with your physician and having an open dialogue is extremely important as you work through what is best for you, whether now or in the future.

THE FREEDOM OF PREVENTIVE MASTECTOMIES

Preventive mastectomies can be emancipating. They allow you to live without looking over your shoulder for cancer all the time. When breast surgeons in New Zealand and Australia asked their patients what made them choose preventive mastectomies for genetic mutations or family history, they said "fear and anxiety."[13]

One major benefit of having preventive mastectomies when there's no cancer diagnosis is that you have control of the timing and can do what works best for your schedule, since they're elective. There are also some guidelines to help figure out the best timing. If a close family member has had breast cancer, it may be a good idea to schedule your surgery before you reach the age of their diagnosis. The timing of events and plans in your own life may also provide a time frame. However, remember that even with the best planning, you may not be able to change your narrative. Waiting is fine, but at some point, cancer can happen, and you never know when that will be.

As we discussed in chapter 2, we're fortunate to have many screening options available, including mammograms, ultrasounds, and MRIs. The primary reason to undergo preventive mastectomies is to prevent breast cancer. Yet the idea that preventive mastectomies allow you to avoid regular scans and biopsies is, for some women, part of the consideration about whether to have prophylactic mastectomies. While most cancers are diagnosed very early through regular screening, there's no guarantee of an early diagnosis, and many women feel that it's easier to avoid it altogether.

Christy was not sure that she would trust mammograms or ultrasounds, since her mother's first cancer was difficult to see on imaging and her second could only be found on an MRI. Christy hated undergoing MRIs. The first time she had one, she thought, *This is what we're making patients go through?* Subjecting herself to forty-five to sixty minutes of loud banging and vibrating noises in a metal tube was difficult. That said, many of our patients in fact find the noise and the solitude in the machine acceptable, sometimes even relaxing. When Rachel has an MRI, she closes her eyes and goes to her happy place—the beach. She doesn't find it to be an overly onerous exam at all. Once again, everyone experiences the procedures and reacts to the stresses differently. That's why those reactions should be a factor in determining what makes the most sense for each individual.

There are other considerations as well. One study of women who had had preventive mastectomies showed that even after two and a half years, 87 percent still had pain in their chests. For 36 percent, it affected their quality of sleep. As many as 75 percent had decreased sexual pleasure. Another 22 percent admitted that the mastectomies had had a negative impact on their daily activities. If those outcomes sound discouraging, consider this. When these same women were asked if they regretted their decision, *none of them* said yes.[14]

We have many patients who are committed to having preventive mastectomies but choose to wait for the right time. It's one of the perks of choosing to have preventive mastectomies without a cancer diagnosis. But keep in mind that none of us can choose when cancer will strike. It can occur anytime. As was discussed earlier, Rachel scheduled preventive mastectomies, but her cancer was diagnosed between the time she scheduled the surgery and the date of the surgery itself.

It's also possible to decide against preventive mastectomies at one time, then change your mind later as new evidence emerges or your situation in life changes. Some wait many years, until they feel that the time is right. After Christy's mother's diagnosis in 2010, Rachel brought up the option of preventive mastectomies and gave Christy the support she needed to make the decision that was right for her. She waited until the following year when the timing was better for work and family. She didn't want to wait until her children were older and more aware of what was happening. The timing was perfect for Christy, and her mother was able to come help while she recovered from surgery, just as Christy had been there for her mother.

The bottom line is, we've never personally seen a woman regret having preventive mastectomies. You will never regret not getting cancer, and if eliminating anxiety about cancer is of primary importance, you will never regret sparing yourself those sleepless nights, knowing full well that this isn't a decision to be made lightly. For many patients, preventive mastectomies provide a welcomed peace of mind.

When making your decisions, it's important to remember that things will never be the same, no matter which path you choose. All options have pros and cons. With breast conservation in one breast, there will likely be asymmetry, and every time you look in the mirror or go to the gym, it will be obvious to you and perhaps others that you were a cancer patient, a stark reminder you may want to avoid. It's also important to know that women often accept their new bodies and become comfortable with them, but if they don't, the asymmetry can often be corrected with plastic surgery, and by law will be covered by insurance. Of course, that does mean another surgery. And the risk of a recurrence or another cancer remains. The older you are, the lower your risk of a new cancer, which is undoubtedly one of the reasons preventive mastectomies are more common in young women.

Christy feels that knowing she will never have breast cancer like her mother did has been an incredible gift. She has never regretted her decision for a single day since her surgery over ten years ago. Rachel had hoped for preventive mastectomies and never having breast cancer, but that isn't what happened. Even with a diagnosis of breast cancer, if Rachel hadn't had bilateral mastectomies twenty-five years ago, she would have had a 50 to 65 percent chance of having another breast cancer by now. Instead, she continues to be at the frontier of early detection, introducing new technologies to improve women's outcomes when diagnosed with breast cancer. She has been instrumental in impacting breast care to underserved communities and educating women across all socioeconomic levels about the importance of risk-based screening, and treasures spending time with her husband, children, and beautiful grandchildren.

We both chose to have mastectomies with reconstruction. We know so many women physicians, indeed other breast cancer physicians, who have made the same choice. We also know breast cancer physicians who opted to have partial mastectomies when their breast cancer was diagnosed. Maybe so many of us do choose mastectomies because we know the consequences of cancer so well. Whatever the reason, we support any woman considering the option of mastectomies, with or without reconstruction. But keep in mind that the decisions that were right for us may be different from the one that's right for you. They're all the right decisions for different women.

Common Questions to Discuss with Your Care Team

How many times have you performed this surgery for this type of breast cancer?

Do you specialize in breast surgery?

Are less invasive treatments available in my case?

Can I keep my nipples? Will I have sensation in my nipples?

How long will I be in the hospital?

Can I talk with other patients of yours who've had a mastectomy?

Will a mastectomy improve my longevity?

How high is my risk of getting this or any other cancer afterward?

What other treatments will I need, and over what period of time?

What are the side effects—shoulder pain? Arm swelling? Lost sensation?

How can I prepare myself emotionally for the surgery?

What are potential complications?

After the surgery, what physical activities will I not be able to do or not be able to do the same way I did before surgery?

CHAPTER 9

Your New Breasts

You've never had more options for reconstructed breasts than you do today. Breast cancer is unlike any other cancer. When you find out you have breast cancer, and need or choose to have a mastectomy, you must make many decisions regarding whether to reconstruct your breast(s) and how, because there are so many options. If you have preventive mastectomies, you have a far better chance of avoiding cancer altogether. There are few, if any, other cancers or organs that have an increased risk of cancer for which there are so many treatment options and so many choices that must be made.

When cancer attacks the pancreas, the lungs, or the liver, part of the organ—sometimes all of it—must be removed. Often we must find ways to compensate for the loss of function that results. Daily insulin injections and digestive enzyme supplements are used to replace the function of the pancreas. There are people who have a genetic mutation that puts them at an extremely high risk of a type of stomach cancer that's very difficult to detect, and who may choose to preventively remove their stomachs. We can reconstruct a stomach, although the function is nothing like the native stomach and patients need to adjust their eating habits to compensate. Women at increased risk for ovarian cancer may choose to have their ovaries and fallopian tubes removed, then take hormone replacement therapy to alleviate menopausal symptoms, as long as they don't have a prior diagnosis of breast cancer.

For many organs, the loss of function is a significant challenge. But thanks to remarkable advances in plastic surgery and reconstructive techniques, as well as new materials and designs and the ever-increasing option of reconstruction with your own tissue (called autologous reconstruction), the options for retaining the appearance of your breasts are excellent.

We still use both saline and silicone implants, but there are more choices than ever. The options for implant shape have expanded; the original round implants are still available, but now you can choose more natural-appearing implants in a teardrop shape if you prefer. Like your original breasts, teardrop implants are fuller at the base and taper toward the top. There are also a wide variety of both smooth and textured implants. Textured implants have a bumpiness to their surface and provide a high-strength cohesive silicone gel that's soft to the touch. The texture on the surface of the implants results in their staying in place and there are actually many different levels of bumpiness to the texture on implants. Smooth round implants provide an even softer feel, but unlike the textured implants, they have a greater tendency to move after placement. They're also more likely to ripple and have a higher contracture rate than textured implants. (Contracture is when your body forms a fibrous capsule around the implant because your immune system sees it as foreign and wants to wall it off from the rest of your body.) The bottom line is, implants come in different shapes with different surface textures.

After implant placement, there may be areas of the breasts that need a bit of "tweaking" to optimize their appearance. In order to achieve that, fat transfer from other parts of the body has become much more versatile and allows us to create more nuance and extra volume to give your breasts a more pleasing appearance.

In some cases, the fat can simply be removed by liposuction from an area where you wish you had less fat in the first place, such as your abdomen or love handles. The plastic surgeon will then inject that fat into the area around your reconstructed breasts to improve the appearance where needed, aiming for the best cosmetic result.[1] More recently, some institutions have begun using fat transfer to reconstruct smaller breasts. However, this procedure is quite new and may require several operations, and some of the possible complications may not yet be fully appreciated.

There are a large number of options for reconstruction using your own tissue, known as autologous reconstruction, that don't require an implant at all. Tissue can be taken from multiple areas in the body and used to reconstruct very natural-looking breasts. The surgery is more involved and usually longer than reconstruction with implants, and often requires microsurgical technique. Therefore, it should be performed by a plastic surgeon with special training and expertise in microvascular breast reconstruction. It's best if the surgeon has both expertise in autologous reconstruction and extra surgical training, such as a fellowship in microsurgery. Although the initial procedure is more involved, the results are lifelong, and don't require replacement or carry associated concerns about rupture or the more recently described infrequent but real concern with implant-associated lymphoma (more about that later in this chapter). Implant-associated lymphoma is a complication of all types of implants, although it's more frequently seen with silicone and textured implants.

Since Kathy didn't have any abdominal fat, our plastic surgeon moved fat from her back, along with the back muscle (latissimus dorsi) to create her new breast. The radiation she had after the mastectomy had hardened the skin, and using the fat and healthier skin from her back to cover the implant allowed us to create more softness and give her the mound to create a beautiful breast. Her new breast doesn't look the same as her healthy breast when she's naked. You can still see the scars from the surgery, and there are visible traces of the changes in her skin caused by radiation. But when she wears clothes—even a bathing suit—you would never know she had been treated for breast cancer. Although it's quite different from her native breast, Kathy is very satisfied with the result.

After she had reconstruction of her nipple, Kathy added the coup de grâce—a new nipple that the plastic surgeon created from her own skin, followed by an attractive, realistic tattoo to simulate the areola.

Plastic surgeons can do extraordinary things. While they do their best to make new breasts look as much like their patients' original ones as possible, there are always differences in appearance, and regardless of the surgeon's skill, you will likely lose sensation in your breasts. It's easier to adjust to your new normal if you know what to expect, and time will help with the adjustment.

Worrying about your lover's reaction to your new breasts is natural, but studies show that a caring partner is most concerned that you're alive and well. They see you as having many parts to love and know you're more than the sum of those parts.[2]

The good news is, your new breasts may look even better than before. That's what happened for us. After having nursed children, we were less than thrilled with the way our breasts looked. And even though we had different types of reconstruction, we both prefer our new breasts. Our new breasts are perkier and more youthful. We know firsthand that while you will need time to adjust to the "new you," you can and hopefully will feel extremely positive about your body and yourself. We understand that the process of coming to this realization and accepting yourself as you are now is different for everyone. It's certainly possible that being in the breast cancer world for our entire careers made the transition easier for us after our own surgeries. For some, it can be incredibly challenging. Know that there are resources such as support groups that can help. The American Cancer Society can be an excellent resource. There's a program called Reach for Recovery where you can be partnered with someone who went through a similar experience to help get you through this challenging time.

Your acceptance of the new you may be particularly positive if you decide to have preventive mastectomies without ever having had breast cancer. Instead of dealing with a potential threat to your life, you've intervened, making a decision that can positively impact your life and that may feel extremely emancipating. You've come to the realization that you can change the narrative of your life with this monumental decision. Even so, every person reacts differently, and the process of and time until acceptance vary widely. Don't hesitate to ask for help from your oncologist, surgeon, or social worker. There are often other resources in your area for you as well.

HOW WE CREATE NEW BREASTS

There are two ways to create new breasts: with implants or with your own tissue. The decision of which option to go with depends on many factors, including the size of your native breasts, your body shape, your available fat, and your personal preference. If you're very thin, you may not have enough fat or other tissue to undergo autologous reconstruction; in these instances, we will recommend an implant for reconstruction. But plastic surgery techniques have improved so much in recent years that it's highly likely that most women can have reconstructed breasts made from their own tissue if that's their preference, especially when the plastic surgeon is very experienced. Curiously enough, doctors find that two years after surgery, women who choose breast reconstruction with their own tissue report greater quality of life satisfaction than those who opt for the simpler procedure associated with an implant.[3]

Regardless of which type of reconstruction a woman chooses, it's important to realize that breast reconstruction often involves multiple procedures. It's rarely completed in one surgery. If both breasts are removed, it's easier to make them match; when only one breast is removed, we almost always recommend additional procedures to improve the appearance and symmetry of the breasts, if the woman wants this. For women having preventive mastectomies, it's not uncommon to first choose the plastic surgeon, and then be referred to the breast surgeon that the plastic surgeon works with the most. For women diagnosed with breast cancer, the choice is more commonly the plastic surgeon that the breast surgeon recommends. Either way, the most important thing is to work with a team that often works together, knows each other, and is there for your best outcome. This isn't the time to cherry-pick your breast surgeon and then your plastic surgeon. If they don't work together regularly, they're not a team, and they aren't the right combination for you.

With breast reconstruction, 20 to 40 percent of patients have complications that require additional surgery. Fortunately, insurance companies are required to cover all stages of breast reconstruction and any procedures necessary to achieve symmetry under the Women's Health and Cancer Rights Act of 1998 (WHCRA). It also requires insurance coverage of bras and prosthetics for women who don't have breast reconstruction, and treatments for the lymphedema that can result from having your lymph nodes removed. While the WHCRA doesn't require insurance companies to cover mastectomies, if a group plan or health insurance issuer covers the mastectomies, then they must also adhere to the WHCRA's requirements.

We will discuss reconstruction with implants and autologous

reconstruction extensively in the following pages. However, as with so many of the choices women faced with either breast cancer or prophylactic mastectomy must make, there are considerations. In this chapter, we'll explore the factors that are helpful to have in mind when making your decision.

NEW BREASTS WITH IMPLANTS

When implants are used for breast reconstruction, they may be placed at the time of the mastectomy. Sometimes final implants cannot be placed at the time of mastectomy, so expanders are placed to stretch the skin to allow for placement of implants at a later time, when the skin is ready. More about this later in this chapter. The advantage to implants is that they're simpler and require a less-involved surgery than reconstruction using your own tissue. But they won't look and feel like your breasts. Mastectomy with implant reconstruction is done under general anesthesia and requires a one- or two-night stay in the hospital and about four weeks off from work for recovery. At our hospital, we offer paravertebral catheters, which provide numbing medication to the chest area for up to a week after surgery. This enables most patients to minimize their need for narcotics for pain relief, and to leave the hospital sooner. On rare occasions, reconstruction is delayed several weeks to allow the skin time to heal. Sometimes an expander is placed as the initial phase of the implant reconstruction. The expander is essentially a deflated implant that can be filled with fluid through a port, or membrane, on its surface. Saline (salt water) is injected gradually to increase the size of the expander, which gently stretches the skin, preparing it for the final implant placement.

This fluid injection is done by someone in the plastic surgery practice, usually a nurse or physician assistant. They will gradually increase the amount of fluid in the expander during sequential office visits, often several weeks apart. Sometime after the final amount of fluid is added to the expander, a same-day surgical procedure is performed to replace the expander with the final implant. The reason you can't simply keep the expander is that it's designed to allow for the gradual insertion of fluid, not to be a long-term device. After the exchange of the expander for the final implant, most women require one to two weeks off from work to heal.

If you choose to have a silicone implant placed for reconstruction, you should know the implant won't last forever. After some time has passed, anywhere between ten and twenty years, the implant will need to be replaced so it doesn't lose its integrity and rupture in your body. You can have ruptured silicone implants without knowing it, so it's recommended that you undergo an MRI every three to five years to have your implants evaluated and ascertain whether they're still intact. If the implants have ruptured, they should be replaced. You can avoid the MRI entirely if you choose saline implants, since they literally deflate if they rupture—something you'd quickly notice! The sterile saline, or salt water, that's in the implant is easily absorbed by your body. You don't need an MRI to determine that. Sometimes implants rupture from a traumatic event, such as a car or bike accident or even a hard fall. If you have any concerns that your silicone implant has ruptured, you can have an MRI to determine this. Importantly, MRIs done to evaluate the integrity of silicone implants do not require the use of a contrast agent like gadolinium, which must be used when MRIs are performed to evaluate for cancer. MRI examination of breast implants is done without any injection or IVs.

Today there are many different types of implants. They're differentiated by whether the implant is filled with saline or silicone. But there are many more considerations. The surface of some implants is smooth, while others have a texture ranging from slightly bumpy to very bumpy. The purpose of the texture is to literally cause mild inflammation so that the body will react to the implant, creating a fibrosis, a shell, around the implant so it will be more likely to stay in place. The fibrosis literally walls the implant off from the rest of the body. Some women, like Christy, prefer to have smooth implants, because they move more readily and feel more comfortable. Others prefer the more natural shape that textured implants provide, but these implants don't move as much as smooth ones do, and may not be as comfortable, especially for women who are very active. There is no perfect implant. If there were, it would be the only one available, but having many varieties speaks to the fact that different implants have different properties that may be preferred by different women. In addition, a more recent consideration is implant-associated lymphoma, which occurs more frequently with textured implants, likely due to the inflammation they cause. (Much more about that in the section on implant risks that follows.)

Ask your plastic surgeon about the different types of implants available. Look at pictures of reconstructions with different sizes, shapes, and types of implants to see what you prefer, and remain as informed as you can be. Don't be reticent to ask the plastic surgeon if they can connect you with a woman who has had the type of implants or autologous reconstruction you're considering so you can talk to them directly, and even feel the implants. Many women are happy to share their experiences with you and to do what they can to help you along your journey. This sisterhood of mastectomies is one of the silver linings of the journey you're on.

Implant Risks

When placing an implant or doing other breast reconstruction, the amount of blood in the skin of the reconstructed breast is very critical. Without adequate blood flow, the skin of the reconstructed breast can potentially die, a difficult complication to treat.

The naked eye isn't adequate to evaluate the blood flow in the mastectomy skin at the time of reconstruction. We don't definitively know how the skin will look until about forty-eight hours after surgery. In our practice, women having bilateral mastectomies spend at least one night in the hospital after surgery, and if there are any concerns about how the skin or reconstruction looks or if their pain isn't sufficiently controlled, they will be offered the option to stay a second night.

A major improvement has been technology that allows the plastic surgeon to check the blood flow in the skin and nipples. We no longer have to rely exclusively on how the skin looks at the time of surgery, which may not accurate. SPY angiography (also called laser-assisted fluorescence) is a relatively new tool that enables plastic surgeons to assess the blood flow in the skin during the reconstruction surgery. A dye, indocyanine green, is injected into a vein in the arm and circulates in the body to indicate the amount of blood flow. A camera using laser angiography visualizes and evaluates the presence of this dye in the blood and makes an accurate determination of the amount of blood going to the skin within minutes. We use this technology for all patients having mastectomies with reconstruction. It takes away the guesswork and concern about how the skin will heal and instead gives us accurate real-time information about how much blood flow there is to the skin, therefore helping us decide how to proceed. Studies have shown that reconstruction with SPY angiography or other advanced methods of assessing the skin during reconstruction results in better outcomes. Therefore, ask your plastic surgeon if they use an intraoperative technique to assess the viability of the skin beyond just the way the it looks. If the technology isn't available in your area or your plastic surgeon doesn't use it, you should feel free to seek a second opinion, but know that many safe and superb reconstructions have been performed without SPY angiography. Just make sure you ask and are fully informed. If the blood flow looks good, we know it's safe to use a permanent implant rather than placing a temporary expander. You may not need the progressive increase in the amount of fluid an expander allows, and if the implant can be placed during the initial surgery, that means one less surgical procedure. However, if the blood flow is inadequate or less than optimal, the skin can become compromised and doesn't do well with the stretching that's needed to insert the final implant at the time of the initial surgery. Therefore, an expander would be placed. Sometimes, even with an expander, the skin may not be healthy after the trauma of the reconstruction, which could result in skin necrosis (skin death). Should that happen, additional procedures to remove the dead skin will be required. The final implants won't be placed until the skin is ready to accept them.

Hyperbaric oxygen therapy (HBOT) is literally sitting or lying in a chamber in which the air you breathe has been concentrated with oxygen. This can increase the amount of oxygen in your blood, which can be helpful in healing skin that has been traumatized by surgery and doesn't have enough oxygen. HBOT might also be recommended to enhance blood flow in the skin and improve its ability to heal. Not every hospital offers HBOT. The treatment takes two hours and sometimes requires either a prolonged hospital stay or a return to the hospital after surgery, but in our experience, women who make use of HBOT are generally able to avoid having skin removed due to necrosis or having other complications from reconstruction. If you have complications related to insufficient blood (and therefore oxygen) to the skin, ask your doctor of HBOT is available in your area.

Implant-Associated Lymphoma

A rare type of lymphoma has been found in one out of a million women with implants. While we can treat this implant-associated lymphoma (IAL) successfully, it requires chemotherapy and the removal of the implants. IAL has been reported with all types of implants, both saline and silicone, smooth and textured. However, studies have shown that it's substantially more frequent in women with textured silicone implants—although it's still rare in these women. Research is ongoing to determine exactly what type of texture is most concerning for IAL and what type of implant is least associated with the disease, so that the safest implants that give the best cosmetic results can be offered to women. Right now we aren't exactly certain which implants are least associated with IAL. Recent studies seem to imply that it may be implants with small bumps in the texture. In fact, some very recent research demonstrates that these slightly bumpy implant surfaces may be associated with lymphoma even less than smooth implants.[4]

When IAL occurs, it's associated with a large amount of fluid surrounding the implant. The way to evaluate if IAL is present is to perform an ultrasound or, more preferably, an MRI to see if there's excess fluid around the implant. The implants that are most frequently associated with the development of this rare lymphoma were removed from the market in 2019, and women with those implants have been informed. It's currently *not* recommended that the implants be removed due to the risk of lymphoma, since this lymphoma is extremely rare, even if you have the type of implants that are most frequently associated with

IAL, since the risk of the surgery is considered greater than the risk of getting IAL. If you ever develop fluid, swelling, or an unfamiliar pain around an implant, see your physician right away to investigate.

Lymphoma resulting from breast implants is so rare that it isn't a reason to not have implant reconstruction, but you should be aware of it, and your plastic surgeon will discuss it at the time of your consultation about reconstruction. It may be a reason to consider autologous reconstruction—but that too has its issues.

Women with implants placed behind the pectoralis (chest wall) muscle experience something known as the "window shade" phenomenon. This describes a situation where every time you raise your arms or use your pectoralis muscle, such as when you're lifting weights, the implant moves. The pectoralis muscle pulls with certain arm movements, causing the reconstruction to have a crease across the implant. While this isn't obvious in clothing, it can be bothersome to women when looking in the mirror without clothing on. Additionally, some women find the movement of the implant itself quite bothersome. Imagine doing lat pull-downs in the gym, and each time you let the bar rise, your implant moves as well. Now that most implants or expanders are being placed in front of the muscle, this is less frequently an issue.

Implant Placement

As mentioned, it's now most common to place the implants in front of the muscle, not behind it. Most patients prefer it. Recovery is easier. There isn't the same tightness of the muscle, and the implant doesn't move during muscle contraction.

The downside is that placing the implant in front of the muscle may mean that the folds that normally occur in the material of the implant encasing the saline or silicone may be visible, because the skin is directly over the implant; these folds or ripples are more visible in thin women. When the implant is behind the muscle, the rippling is hidden. Rippling makes the reconstruction look less natural and more like an implant. It occurs more often with smooth implants. It's most obvious when looking in the mirror, but it can also be noticeable for some women when wearing bathing suits and sometimes even through clothing.

One possible solution is fat transfer. As with breast reconstruction, a plastic surgeon can use liposuction to move fat from elsewhere in the body to cover the rippling and contour of the breast. All these additional surgical procedures to improve the appearance and feel of the implant are performed in the operating room under general anesthesia as same-day procedures. Some women choose to undergo these procedures, while others are sufficiently pleased with their reconstruction, even with some rippling, and choose to not undergo additional procedures to improve the appearance of the implant. Once again, there are so many choices, and the right choice for an individual woman is very personal.

When Christy had her first surgery in 2011, the option of having implants placed in front of the muscle was not available, so hers were placed behind. Direct-to-implant reconstructions were also not offered back then, so she had reconstruction with expanders. This afforded her the added advantage that the gradual increase in size of the expanders allowed her to actually see what the final size of her implants would look like, and she chose the stopping point when the expander size was what she wanted. However, expanders are tight and very hard. Christy described the feeling of the expanders as bricks under her skin—exactly as her patients had described them. Of course, this feeling changes when the expanders are switched out for the final implants.

When Christy underwent the exchange of the expanders for her final implants, she found the surgery to be very tolerable. She went home the same day and resumed her normal activities, aside from jogging, within a week. In two weeks, she was jogging again.

Christy loved how the implants felt, even though they were nothing like her original breasts. For the first year, it would often feel like she was always wearing a bra even when she wasn't because of the tightness, but over time she got used to the implants. The numbness improved as well, but sensation in the nipples never returned. There's some rippling since she's thin, but it isn't noticeable, even when she's wearing a bathing suit, so she doesn't find it bothersome. Christy does have the "window shade" effect, but no one notices but her, and she has learned to ignore it. It isn't painful; it just looks and sometimes feels funny because the implants move with certain hand and arm movements, such as when she opens a jar.

In early 2021, Christy had to have her implants replaced due to a rupture of the left implant. While this sounds alarming, it's not. In fact, she didn't know it had been ruptured for over a year. After a fall in 2020 that had her concerned about her right implant, she had an MRI. Interestingly, the MRI showed that the right implant was fine but the left implant had ruptured and needed to be replaced. She was offered the option of having the muscle pulled down and the new implants placed in front of the muscle. This is a great option, but because it's a more involved surgery and Christy wanted the quickest recovery possible, she chose to have the new implants placed behind the muscle where the old ones had been so she could get back to work within the week.

For women who have tightness due to implants placed behind the muscle, the option of repositioning them in front of the muscle is possible and may be a good one, as long as they know the procedure is more involved than just replacing the implants that are already there. Women who have implants behind the muscle that need to be replaced should talk to their plastic surgeons about the possibility of having the new implants placed in front of the muscle. Plastic surgeons are constantly working on options to improve results for patients, and this is just one example.

RECONSTRUCTED BREASTS WITH YOUR OWN TISSUE

When you use your own tissue for breast reconstruction, the result looks and feels more like a natural breast. After all, it's your own tissue. There are other advantages of autologous reconstruction, which include that fact that you will never need to replace the tissue (as you would with an implant), no follow-up imaging is required, it doesn't move when you do, and there's no risk of lymphoma from the reconstruction. These sound great, but there's always a cost, and the cost for autologous reconstruction is more extensive surgery.

The disadvantages are the longer time in the operating room, longer stay in the hospital, longer recovery, and additional incisions in the places on your body from which the tissue was taken (the donor sites). Just as with implant reconstruction, the reconstructed breasts are generally numb, but many women describe increased sensation with time, although never back to what it was before surgery. And as we mentioned earlier, you may need to have further surgeries to achieve the desired cosmetic result, although women are often sufficiently pleased with the initial reconstruction that additional surgery is not needed.

As you make your decision, it may help to think of it in terms of what the cost of your choice is—that is, which parts are the most difficult for you and when will you have to do them?

With your own tissue, the cost is immediate: longer surgery and slower recovery.

With implants, the cost comes later: continued surveillance imaging with MRI, implant movement with arm movement, and the very small but still present risk of implant-associated lymphoma.

If you're one of the women for whom MRI is very difficult, having implants may feel like it defeats the purpose of your preventive mastectomy. You'll still have to have regular MRIs, although they will be every three to five years instead of every year, and the study doesn't require the injection of contrast (gadolinium) required for MRIs done to evaluate for cancer. All this needs to be considered when deciding what type of reconstruction to opt for.

Although it was a longer, more difficult surgery, Rachel chose to do autologous reconstruction with her own tissue. After double mastectomies, fat and muscle were taken from her transverse rectus abdominis myocutaneous (TRAM) area, or lower abdomen (the most commonly used site for tissue harvest for autologous breast reconstruction), to create her new breasts. The abdominal muscle and fat replaced the breast, and the muscle provided the blood flow to the fat. The reconstruction used the tissue from her abdomen, so an added benefit was that she ended up with a tummy tuck, too. The tissue needed for the reconstruction was taken from an area where there was "too much" tissue, particularly after two pregnancies, one with twins. Although Rachel would not have chosen to undergo a tummy tuck on its own, she was certainly happy to have it as part of the reconstruction.

For Rachel, "one and done" was very important. She didn't want to replace implants in the future. She's extremely happy with the reconstruction not only because her breasts look and feel natural but also because when her weight changes, the size of her breasts does as well.

Once the reconstruction was done, she no longer had to worry about future surgeries or MRIs, as she would have with implants. The downside is that because some of her abdominal muscles were used, part of her core musculature is missing. Although a mesh was inserted to help restore strength and stability to the abdomen, it's not as if her core muscles are intact. Nevertheless,

Rachel can do any activity she could before the surgery, including sit-ups, and any activity she would like to do. Today, no muscle is used in reconstruction with abdominal tissue, so this is no longer a consideration. Today, the tissue taken from the abdomen to reconstruct breasts doesn't include any muscle, so the core musculature remains intact. The techniques used in reconstruction are constantly improving!

There are even excellent options for re-creating a nipple and areola if they have been removed during surgery. The nipple tattooing available now is so advanced that some tattoo artists can make a 3D-looking nipple with ink alone. The ability to make a flat object seem 3D has been part of the art world for thousands of years and is called trompe l'oeil (French for "deceive the eye"). It literally makes flat images look convincingly three-dimensional. There are some tattoo artists who specialize in tattooing the nipple, like the Vinnie Myers Team in Maryland. There may be similar places near you. Ask your plastic surgeon about the availability of trompe l'oeil nipple tattooing.

Abdominal Fat

There are different ways to use abdominal tissue to reconstruct breasts following mastectomy. One, called the transverse rectus abdominis muscle (TRAM) flap, was popular for tissue reconstruction in the 1990s. However, with TRAM reconstruction, part of the rectus abdominus muscle (the abs) is taken, and there can be a biomechanical deficit. Advances in breast reconstruction with abdominal muscle have led to the development of deep inferior epigastric perforator (DIEP) flap reconstructions. Like TRAM reconstructions, the abdominal tissue is used, but only the fat is taken; the abdominal musculature is left intact. Therefore, you get the benefit of a flatter stomach without losing any function. In the past, women who had autologous reconstruction using abdominal muscle and fat were at risk of developing abdominal hernias. Today, that's not a significant concern, because the abdominal muscles are preserved.

If you're considering autologous reconstruction with the use of abdominal tissue, be certain you have a DIEP flap reconstruction. Women should not undergo TRAM flaps anymore in order to preserve abdominal wall function. With a DIEP flap, the plastic surgeon connects the blood vessels that supply the abdominal fat to the blood vessels in the chest using a microscope, a highly technical surgical technique called microvascular surgery.

Naturally, this complex surgery takes longer than an implant reconstruction. The hospital stay is around three to five days. In some institutions, the first day or two may be spent in the intensive care unit (ICU) for appropriate monitoring. However, this isn't always the case, and appropriately trained nursing on a regular floor can be sufficient. Again, many differences are found around the country. Most women will require eight weeks to recuperate from this surgery. However, some might well be ready to return sooner.

Plastic surgeons who perform DIEP flaps must be trained in microvascular surgery, so if you pursue this option, you absolutely want to find a very experienced plastic surgeon who regularly performs DIEP reconstructions. And be certain to ask the difficult questions: "Do you do DIEP reconstructions? Do you have specialty training in microvascular surgery? How many DIEP flaps have your performed? How many in the past year? What is your success rate?" If anyone tells you they have a 100 percent success rate, go elsewhere. Nothing in medicine is ever 100 percent!

You always want a team that works together. This work is like conducting a symphony. The harmony and familiarity of working together as a team will increase the likelihood of the best outcome. So don't insist on *your* plastic surgeon working with *your* breast surgeon. Think of it as *your team*, and *your outcome* will be the best it can be.

After Betty Jones had a left mastectomy in 2006, she needed radiation because there was cancer in many of her lymph nodes. At the time, she chose to replace her breast with an implant, but she never liked it. Radiation had hardened the implant, so it was always uncomfortable, and she never liked how high it was compared to her healthy breast.

We discussed the option of having her implant replaced using a DIEP reconstruction. At first she was hesitant to have another surgery, but she ultimately decided to do it. The implant was removed and replaced with her abdominal fat. Now her breasts are more symmetric. Not only does the reconstructed breast feel much more natural to her but she also loves the added benefit of having a flat abdomen.

Donor Sites

Tissue can be taken from many areas of your body to reconstruct your breasts. Generally, the first area that's used is the abdominal tissue, as described earlier. However, many areas of the body can be used, and this section describes alternative options to abdominal tissue. The premise is fundamentally the same, but the procedure varies, depending on where the tissue is taken and whether the muscle is taken with it.

When the fat tissue taken along with a small flap of the gracilis muscle in the inner thigh, the procedure is called a transverse upper gracilis (TUG) flap. It's one of the better locations to remove tissue, since four muscles in that area work together to move the thigh inward and a small piece of one of them can be removed without noticeably altering the function of the thigh. The downside is that only a small piece of muscle can be taken, so TUG flaps tend to be smaller than flaps taken from other parts of the body. There's also a tendency toward swelling in the groin and lower leg afterward.[5]

It's also possible to remove your buttock love handles in order to create new breasts. This is an option with obvious cosmetic appeal. We call them gluteal artery perforator (GAP) flaps, based on the name of the blood vessel that runs through the area from the upper buttocks.[6]

Both TUG and GAP flaps are excellent options for patients who don't have enough abdominal fat for DIEP flaps or who have had prior abdominal surgery and are not candidates for DIEP flaps. They're ideal for patients who have extra tissue in the buttock or upper thigh regions and small breasts.

Because they require specialized training—not only in microvascular surgery but also in the complicated reconstruction itself—TUG and GAP flaps are not offered at every hospital, but most plastic surgeons will know the best place to go for these flaps. The hospital stay and recovery time are similar to those for DIEP reconstructions.

Although Karen Smith was a good candidate for TUG flaps, she was undecided. She elected to have bilateral mastectomies after being diagnosed with early-stage breast cancer. Since her sister was being treated for metastatic disease at the time, the mastectomies were an easy decision for her, but deciding on the type of reconstruction was more difficult.

One thing she did know was that she absolutely did not want to have implants. She decided that she would use her own tissue, but she didn't have enough abdominal fat to do DIEP flaps. She did have enough thigh fat for TUG flaps, but she was warned that even though she didn't have large breasts, her new breasts would be even smaller. TUG reconstructions often don't provide enough tissue to fill out an entire breast. We explained to Karen that her breasts would likely be smaller, and that she would likely require additional procedures to fill in the top of her breasts with fat grafting if she wanted fuller-looking breasts. She decided that this option was best for her, and she was fine with the results.

The most difficult part of her recovery was her thighs. Sitting was uncomfortable after surgery. This is a common side effect, since the incisions cut through the gluteal creases, where the buttocks meet the thighs—exactly the area that comes into play when we sit.

While Karen knows that she has the option of doing additional fat grafting and that insurance will cover the cost of the procedures, she isn't interested in any more surgery, since her reconstructed breasts are not much smaller than her original ones were. In addition, she's too busy to take the necessary time off to recover from fat grafting, which can take one to two weeks.

Latissimus Dorsi Flaps

Another common area to derive tissue for new breasts is from the latissimus dorsi, the large muscle from the middle and lower back that connects the bones of your upper arms to your spine. For those who work out, these muscles are commonly referred to as the lats.

Latissimus dorsi flaps (LDFs) are now performed less frequently, but because they tend to have fewer complications afterward, they can be an excellent reconstructive choice for women who want to avoid the increased risks of the other options, and plastic surgeons don't require specialized training to do them. They're also a good option for women who want to avoid implants but are not good candidates for longer surgeries such as DIEP or TUG/GAP reconstructions.

LDFs are also used for women who have had prior radiation but need an implant, since they can cover the implant and reduce the risk of implant contracture. The flaps can also be used for partial breast reconstructions for women who have asymmetry after breast conservation surgery and radiation. The surgery is generally longer than implant reconstructions but faster than DIEP reconstructions. It doesn't require a stay in the ICU—just two or three nights in the hospital, followed by four to six weeks for recovery.

The main complaint from these reconstructions is tightness in the back and the large scar, which is visible in gowns with low-cut backs and in bathing suits. There isn't any change in physical activity after recovery from surgery.

When Marjorie Longfellow was in her seventies, she developed cancer in her right breast. It was her third round of breast cancer. Years before, when she developed cancer in her left breast, she had a mastectomy followed by TRAM reconstruction. Later, she was diagnosed with cancer in her right breast and had a partial mastectomy (breast conservation) including radiation. She was never happy with how that breast looked, since it was so much smaller than her reconstructed breast. By the time she developed another cancer in her right breast, she knew she would have to undergo a mastectomy. It was her chance to give her right breast the look and feel of her left breast. So she decided to undergo a flap reconstruction.

Since she was in her seventies, we didn't want to put her through the longer surgery of a TUG reconstruction. Instead, we recommended a lat flap. She had enough fat in her back to do it, and her recovery was relatively straightforward. She was in the hospital for two days and back to all her normal activities in six weeks.

Having so many different reconstruction options allows us to find the best approach for each patient.

Nipple and Areola

If you didn't have nipple-sparing mastectomies and choose to have your nipples reconstructed, several months after you have your reconstruction, you will come into the hospital as an outpatient for the reconstruction of your nipple and areola. Remember that this doesn't re-create sensation, just the cosmetic appearance of the nipple. It's noteworthy that you can certainly have your breast reconstructed without the additional surgery of nipple reconstruction if you so choose.

Plastic surgeons first re-create your nipple from the skin remaining after your mastectomy. Sometimes they can even do "nipple sharing," in which part of the nipple on your healthy breast is used to re-create a nipple. Then, several weeks after that, an ordinary tattoo of the new nipple and surrounding tissue can create an image of the areola that's so convincing that it will be hard to tell it's a tattoo.

Like Kathy Daniels, whom you'll recall from the beginning of this chapter, you can also choose the very popular option of a 3D tattoo that looks like a nipple and areola. Although the surface will be smooth, the look is remarkably convincing. There are two notable advantages to this. One is that you avoid having another surgery to re-create your nipples. The other is that you no longer need to wear a bra to cover the protrusion of your nipples.

Many of our patients love the Vinnie Myers Team in Maryland. Vinnie was among the first to develop the 3D tattoo to re-create nipples. He has set aside a special room in his tattoo parlor for women wishing to have a new nipple and areolar complex. It's incredible to see how real and three-dimensional these tattoos are when they're done by a team as talented as Vinnie's. Our patients call him "Vinnie the tattoo artist." Now there are tattoo artists and plastic surgeons throughout the country who offer the procedure.

DELAYS

Immediate reconstruction following a mastectomy will give you the best look in the end. The skin of the breast is preserved during the mastectomy, along with the nipples (if you don't have cancer that involves the nipples), so that gives you an advantage. But some women must delay reconstruction for six to twelve months for medical reasons, until after their initial mastectomies and cancer treatments are completed. In some cases, reconstruction must be delayed due to the extent of disease, the need for radiation, or the skin not receiving enough oxygen from blood. Although you can still get good results even when surgery is delayed, doing immediate reconstruction provides the best results.

Katrina Dickenson didn't want to delay her reconstruction, but she was diagnosed with left breast cancer in April 2020 in the early days of the COVID-19 pandemic, when many hospitals were not even offering surgery for cancer patients. Fortunately, at the George Washington University Hospital in Washington, DC, where we work, we were allowed to continue to operate on cancer patients. But for several weeks when the number of patients admitted for COVID-19 was high, breast reconstructions were classified as elective surgeries and could not be performed due to the overwhelming need of resources for COVID patients. We didn't know how long it would be before we could offer reconstruction.

Since Katrina, fifty-five, had cancer in more than one area of her breast, we recommended that she have a mastectomy, but told her we couldn't offer reconstruction due to the high COVID numbers. She didn't want to delay surgery and was less concerned about reconstruction than removing the cancer. After the mastectomy, she wore a bra with a prosthetic on the left side.

Once we were able to resume breast reconstructions, Katrina was not eager to go through several more surgeries and was considering delaying even further. We encouraged her to meet with a plastic surgeon to discuss her options. A DIEP reconstruction was a good option for her because she had enough abdominal fat to re-create the breast. She was pretty sure it would be the best option for her, but wanted to wait until we knew more about how the pandemic would progress. She had a simple mastectomy without reconstruction and used a prosthesis with a mastectomy bra. Finally, a year later, she had a DIEP reconstruction, and she loves her new breast.

Every woman prioritizes different aspects of reconstruction. While Katrina dreaded the thought of more surgeries enough to delay her reconstruction, Joanne Carlson was very motivated to have reconstruction at the time of her mastectomy. Some women are motivated by a "one and done" approach, where the major concern for others is achieving the best cosmetic result possible. Some women are focused on the most minimal surgery, whereas others make choices strongly influenced by having reconstruction without the need for future imaging or concerns with implant rupture. As with so much, the "best" solution is different for every woman.

After she was diagnosed with breast cancer on the right at the age of forty-five, Joanne had mastectomies on both sides and opted for implants to create her new breasts. She was treated with chemotherapy, followed by radiation therapy on right side.

Then her right implant got infected and had to be removed. It's uncommon, but unfortunately can happen. Afterward, she needed time to recover from the infection before reconstruction could be offered. While she was waiting, she wore a bra with a silicone prosthesis (the cost of which was covered by insurance) so her breasts would look the same in clothes.

Because Joanne had had radiation, her skin was hard and would not stretch, so we had to use abdominal fat to reconstruct her breast instead of another implant. She didn't have a lot of abdominal fat, so we warned her that she would need more procedures to make her right breast symmetric with the left one. Liposuction from other parts of her body for fat grafting to increase the size of her right breast would be necessary to achieve symmetry. Joanne didn't mind having these additional procedures. What was critical to her was that her breasts were as symmetric as possible and that all the procedures were covered by insurance. Not counting the removal of the implant, it took four surgeries to match her right breast to her left breast. Since that time, she has remained cancer-free and is satisfied with her cosmetic results.

This chapter discussed numerous approaches to breast reconstruction. One thing is certain, regardless of the type of reconstruction you undergo—your reconstructed breasts will neither look nor feel like your native breasts. However, the outcomes are often more than acceptable, and most women are pleased with their choices. In addition, it's important to realize that there is no one "right" decision. That's why it's so important to understand the implications of each option; the right decision is different for different women, and information is the best way to discover what is right for you.

Reconstruction has its challenges, but in our practice we find that most women are generally pleased with it. We consider it vital that breast reconstruction is performed by an experienced team of breast and plastic surgeons who work together regularly and are very familiar with each other. Over the years, we've seen the benefits of this close relationship again and again. There's no substitute for a great, cohesive team.

With new breasts, the elephant in the room is inevitably how your sex life will be impacted. While change and healing always take time, many of our patients report stronger, more precious, and more loving relationships after going through these changes. (This will be discussed more in chapter 11.) It has every potential to draw you closer to those you love. We feel fortunate that this has been our experience, and we hope it will be yours as well.

Common Questions to Discuss with Your Care Team

What are the pros and cons of immediate versus delayed reconstruction?

What are my options for reconstruction?

Are there different recovery periods for women who undergo implant reconstruction versus reconstruction with their own tissue?

How many procedures will I need to have before the reconstruction is complete?

Are there any new types of reconstruction I should consider, including clinical trials?

Can you show me photos of your patients' typical results?

Do you have a patient who underwent a procedure similar to the one I anticipate having that I could talk to?

How many reconstruction procedures do you perform every year?

How many reconstructions of the type I've chosen have you performed over the past year?

Which plastic surgeon should I consult to decide what my next steps are?

Are there potential problems that I should be prepared for?

Will a tissue flap leave scars or other changes in the area the tissue was taken from?

How long do breast implants last?

What are the odds that an implant will leak or cause other problems?

What kinds of complications commonly occur during reconstruction?

What kinds of changes to my reconstruction can I expect in the coming years?

Does aging have an impact on breast reconstruction?

CHAPTER 10

How Your Loved Ones Can Help

In our own lives, our spouses have stood by us through all the challenges we've faced. As daughters, we've supported our mothers while they had cancer. As mothers, we've shared our daughters' concerns about their increased risk of breast cancer and the impact of cancer on their lives and future. Our many dear friends and close relatives are an essential part of our lives. Without them, every day would be more difficult and, indeed, sometimes intolerable. And it goes without saying that we've stood by and supported our many patients as they went through their breast cancer journeys.

Every person, whether male or female, is deeply impacted by breast cancer—even if they themselves or their immediate family members haven't had breast cancer. With one in eight American women having breast cancer in their lifetime, there is no workplace, house of worship, community group, or family where someone isn't affected by breast cancer. In communities with even higher rates of breast cancer, such as Ashkenazi Jewish communities and communities of color, this is even more evident.

Nearly a quarter million women in the US will be diagnosed with breast cancer this year, which means that many spouses, partners, friends, and loved ones will become caregivers. We now know that how your loved ones and broader social connections respond to your diagnosis makes a significant difference in your recovery. Nowhere is this truer than the impact of breast cancer on the life partner of a person who has been diagnosed with breast cancer. The social, sexual, and nonmedical reaction of a woman to breast cancer is a critical part of her recovery and readjustment after treatment, and it's markedly different in every person, at every age, and at every stage of life. This is equally true for women at increased risk of breast cancer and how it affects their lives.

As the significant other, parent, child, relative, or close friend, there are so many things you can do while your loved one goes through the process of deciding to have mastectomies or managing the treatments necessary for a cancer diagnosis. As healthcare providers, we're often so focused on our patients that we sometimes don't address the needs of those who are there to support them. But because our spouses have been through the breast cancer journey with us, we've had an inside view of what they were going through. As daughters, we've supported our mothers, and as mothers, we're plagued by the consequences our cancer diagnoses and treatments have had on our children. This chapter deals with the needs of loved ones and provides guidance for how they might best help. This won't be able to address every single situation, but we hope that by including our stories and those of some of our patients, you may find some information that your loved ones will find helpful.

SUPPORT

When someone you love is diagnosed with breast cancer, so many decisions must be made: What kind of surgery, where, when, even how? Will there be chemotherapy, radiation, or medications? Eventually all these decisions will be made, but the beginning of the journey is filled with overwhelming amounts of information as well as uncertanties that can be confusing. Many key areas of support are necessary. The decision-making process is often one of the most difficult parts of a cancer journey for both the patient and their loved ones. As a supporter, it's important to look for ways to be an advocate. Volunteer to or help identify who will take responsibility for keeping everything organized during the seemingly endless doctor's appointments while providing emotional support. Communication is key during this time, so listen and give your loved one space if necessary. Reassure her that you're completely supportive of any decision she makes. If you don't necessarily agree with the choices she makes, at least keep the lines of communication open and listen to her. It's essential that you understand and respect her reasoning. The needed help that loved ones provide during the recovery process can be different for different women. Throughout the course of treatment, there will likely be times when being there for her will mean everything—and it's equally likely that there will be times when the presence of others is a burden. During treatment, intimacy may need to be adjusted, but once fully recovered, the hope is to maintain the intimacy and affection that was there previously, and often perhaps improve it. The critical thing to remember is to communicate: ask questions, pay attention to signals, and remember that things are likely to change often as treatment progresses. Needs will shift, and the best way to offer support is to ask.

It's equally important to realize that caretakers and those in support networks have needs as well. This is an emotionally difficult time for them, and they, too, must have the realization that no matter how hard they try, they won't be able to do everything that's needed, or always say the right thing. And indeed, there may be life partners who find this time in their lives is overwhelming. They simply cannot withstand the unimaginable stress of a cancer diagnosis and treatment in the person who has always been there to support and care for them. How can the tables be turned so quickly? The important thing is that the lines of communication remain open so that everyone—the person undergoing cancer treatment and all those around them—understands what is expected, what is possible, and, indeed, what is not possible. Everyone will try to do the best they can, but what's best and what's possible will not only be different for everyone but will change. No one will be able to do the right thing all the time. In fact, the "right" words and actions will change. It's important to remember this during what will undoubtedly be an incredibly stressful time of life.

OPEN COMMUNICATION

There are so many things all of us can do in the face of cancer, whether we're supporting those we love or being supported by them. Open communication is key and essential in relationships between people with cancer and those who care about them. How we communicate is deeply influenced by our personalities, as well as our cultures and upbringing.

Some relationships grow much stronger during a crisis that taps into so many primal anxieties, hopes, and fears. With the pressures of cancer or the possibility of prophylactic mastectomies looming, communication with your loved ones is critical.

It's important for the person with cancer to be communicative and let those around them know what they're comfortable talking about and how they would like to discuss issues. Some advice for the cancer patient or the person considering prophylactic mastectomies is to tell their loved ones how much they want to share. Virtually everyone will need someone to help them think through the many difficult decisions that must be made. As the support person, you won't have all the answers. What you do have is a shoulder your loved one can lean on. The most important thing is that you empathize. You won't be able to solve the problems at hand or even fully understand them. You just need to let your loved one know you're with them and always there supporting them.

As the support person, ask if you can help with research regarding major treatment decisions. It can be helpful to have a point person for finding second opinions or additional information to help make an important choice. This is especially true because the support person is one step removed from the patient themselves, undoubtedly allowing consideration of different options. However, if the patient is comfortable with her care team and doesn't want additional opinions or research, go with her to her appointments as her scribe and take extensive notes. So much information is provided during doctor's visits that it can be overwhelming, and that information may well require additional time and additional consideration to come to the decision that's best for her.

Every person and every family have different coping mechanisms and styles of communication. No matter how you've interacted with one another in the past, it's crucial at this time in your life to talk about needs and emotions with honesty and sincerity. Because we're trying our best to help those we love, we naturally worry about how to best deal with the situation.

Listening is as important as talking. The person who's going through cancer will let you know, often in subtle ways, how they're best comforted. And many loved ones, as much as they desire to help and show their support, will feel like they don't know what to say. Talking about cancer is hard. Should they deal with cancer directly or avoid the topic? Do you try to get your loved one's mind off the difficulties or focus on the positives and minimize the negatives? Talk about how proud you are of her strength and will. Reassure her that you will get through this together, and perhaps your relationship will be even stronger as a result. Cherish the extra time that you spend together. Ask how she's feeling, what she's thinking, and what considerations are going into the difficult decisions that accompany a breast cancer diagnosis. Many discussions will be repeated, but this reconsideration is going to be critical and is part of the sequential steps required to get to the final decisions.

CHANGES TO RELATIONSHIPS

Whatever the outcome of this journey, the changes to your expectations of life, your daily experiences, your body, and your future are profound, both for you and for your loved ones. Dealing with that is quite enough, but you should also prepare yourself for the fact that the changes you're experiencing will unavoidably create both psychological and physical changes in your relationships.

If you have young children, you may notice they're displaying different emotions and behavior. These shifts won't always be rational, to them or to you. It's not uncommon for young children to become clingy or impulsive, or for older children to become angry or distant. Encourage them to talk about what they're feeling. Reassure them that they will always be loved. It's never a bad idea to consider counseling, particularly if they aren't willing to open up to you. Don't hesitate to reach out to your child's pediatrician for support and advice. Ask the social worker or nurse navigator at your oncologist's practice for support resources. For some, counseling can be an outstanding resource to get through this time. For others, navigating this process without counseling is the way to move forward. The journey is different for everyone. The important thing to remember is to seek help if and when you need it. Those around you want to help and the resources available are different in every location, but *never* hesitate to ask.

The dynamics in relationships can shift in awkward ways after a breast cancer diagnosis or a positive test for genetic mutation. We all fulfill certain roles for one another. When someone has always relied on you to care for them, they may struggle with moving into the role of caregiver. It's not uncommon for the patient to be strong or stoic, and the loved one to be struggling with the diagnosis. It may be difficult for the patient to give up the roles she normally occupies in the household, and it can be stressful for a loved one to have to take on those responsibilities.

Apart from psychological changes, your own physical needs will change, at least temporarily, during your treatment and recovery. You're likely to experience changes in energy level, appetite, sleep patterns, mobility, and desire for intimacy. Talk with your physician about what you can expect, then discuss the limitations and possible solutions with those who are there to help.

It goes without saying that the physical changes that come with either a breast cancer diagnosis and treatment or prophylactic mastectomy are profound. Every woman deals with the physical changes and the mourning for their "old self" differently. However, try to help your loved one with the insight needed to adjust to these difficult changes. There are many support groups, often local, that deal with the body changes that occur with the surgeries necessary for treating or preventing cancer. Don't hesitate to seek out these resources for the one you love. No one will understand her needs better than you can, so be there not only to support her directly but also to identify local resources that can help with the body change readjustment, along with the enormous emotional changes she will experience.

One excellent national resource is the American Cancer Society (ACS, cancer.org). They have many resources, including Reach to Recovery, where a woman is partnered with a woman who has gone through similar treatment and can provide support. There are also numerous, and excellent, local support groups. If the support group or counseling you need isn't available directly from the ACS, they can direct you to local resources that can help.

WAYS TO HELP

Inevitably, your loved ones and friends will ask what they can do to help. When they say, "Let me know if you need anything," most of them mean it, and would drop what they're doing to help. Most likely, as you're going through this difficult time, friends, family, and colleagues think about you more than you know. Whether they're showing up at your door or not, a tacit part of the circle of love surrounds you.

Appointing someone to share medical updates with your loved ones and community will relieve you of having to repeat the information again and again. Email updates or texts with those in your circle will be of great benefit.

Too often people undergoing major challenges are reluctant to ask friends for help or simply don't know what they'll need. It's far better to allow your loved ones to show you how much they care than to leave them wishing they could do more or even turning away their heartfelt efforts to be supportive.

Millions of people have been through this before you and have already discovered what was helpful for them. Here are some things that have been appreciated by others who have gone through what you're going through now. Use these lists to make suggestions when your friends ask what they can do.

The Basics

- Always call first. Don't just show up at the door.
- Make calls or visits short and frequent, rather than long and irregular.
- Know that plans might be canceled at the last minute or even cut short, if the patient isn't feeling well. Don't take it personally. It's not you. It's the illness.

What to Do

- **Care packages.** Put together a little bundle of joy filled with books, movies, snacks, comfy pajamas, favorite obsessions—whatever might be fun or distracting.
- **Errands.** Little things may be much harder for a while. A friend who offers to pick up the house, get medications, or give rides to doctor's appointments is a boon. With so many services available today, it may also be worth offering to schedule a visit from a home cleaning service or helping to set up deliveries.
- **Childcare.** Providing a quiet afternoon without kids is an easy way to help a lot.
- **Care team.** Friends banding together is one of the best solutions. Forming a phone chain for regular calls or for dropping off home-cooked meals is ideal. One group of friends put together a book where each of them wrote about the qualities they admired about their sick friend, complete with photographs and happy memories.
- **Checking in.** Letting the patient know that you're thinking of her is one of the best things you can offer as a friend. Frequent texts or calls, as long as they're quick and lighthearted, make the world feel like a happier, safer place. Responding quickly when the patient reaches out helps, too.
- **Asking what the patient prefers.** Whether she prefers to have

loved ones accompany her to the doctor and take notes, or prefers to retreat and recover on her own, her loved ones can accommodate that choice. Ask her what's best today, as her needs may change. This is one of the areas that can really improve your communication with a loved one who's going through treatment.

- **Special circumstances.** Bringing a casserole may be the traditional thing to do, but during cancer treatment, she may be nauseous and want to avoid food. With a weakened immune system, flowers may not always be appropriate, either. Strong scents or perfumes can be overwhelming when you're going through chemotherapy. These are considerations you may not expect. But it doesn't have to be a mystery. Communication can keep things on track.

What to Say

Cancer is scary. Those who have never helped a loved one through a serious health challenge may have no idea how to talk about it. Keep in mind that someone who's upbeat and optimistic may not be denying the facts. With breast cancer, there's generally good reason for hope, and the person you're supporting likely has learned that from her physicians. Everyone copes with stress in different ways, and indeed, at different times you and the one you love will feel differently. Expect to cycle through emotions that may range from sheer optimism to absolute dread. They're all normal. What is important is to talk about how you feel—and how those around you feel, understanding that it's a dynamic process with an enormous range of emotions. Seize the moments of positive outlook but equally accept the "downs." All these emotions are part of the diagnosis/treatment/healing process.

For the patient, be quick to let your friends know that no matter how sick you feel or frightened you are at any given moment, you haven't lost your sense of humor just because you have cancer. Loved ones who can laugh together, even in the darkest moments, are indispensable. Having a trusted resource you can laugh with and confide in, no matter how you're feeling, will profoundly ease the burden while you're on this difficult path. But be assured that crying together is normal and can be a source of strength. Everyone cries during this period—both the patient and the people who love them.

Whether you're the patient or the caretaker, it's important to always remember to be cognizant of the patient's needs. We need to be sensitive to helping the patient avoid feeling like they have to comfort the people around them, instead of the opposite, when the healthy experience of sharing honest emotions starts to tip into something else. Of course, sometimes the woman may want to support those around her, especially if she has always been a primary caretaker and support system for those she loves. How do you tell the difference? We really can't give you a road map for this, since everyone is different and every relationship is different. However, some basic tips are:

- Be available to listen. Let her know that you're available anytime.
- Let her know you're available to talk or take a call whenever she needs.
- Be yourself.
- Let her know you care. Often during these trying times, this reminder is critical.

What you shouldn't do:
- Don't share every new treatment or cure that you heard about. Many are not yet available, and many won't be applicable to her specific treatment.

- Don't burden her with your worries or fears.
- Don't share how she should be healthier with lifestyle changes. She already has cancer and has enough to deal with at this time of her life.
- Don't tell her to be "positive." She's doing the best she can.
- AND MOST OF ALL: Don't share horror stories of your or someone else's experiences with cancer care. That's the last thing anyone wants to hear, and equally important to remember, everyone's experiences with cancer therapy are different. Some women continue to work, travel, and have some normalcy. Others are completely out of commission. Everyone is different, so stay upbeat and skip the horror stories. They help no one.

While you're recovering between treatments, you may not have the energy to engage in all the social distractions you would normally enjoy with your loved ones. This may be an ideal time to grow closer to the people you love by talking more about your lives. As close as you are to one another, there may be stories you haven't mentioned yet, or deeply held thoughts, hopes, and fears you haven't shared.

PARENTS AND CHILDREN

The bond between parents and children can be so strong that it can be difficult to see the situation objectively, whether it's a child supporting a parent with cancer or, perhaps more challenging, a parent supporting a child through the difficult journey of cancer or prophylactic mastectomy. Watching people you love so dearly endure decisions and treatments like these can be hard to bear.

Parents supporting a child going through the diagnosis of breast cancer or a decision to have mastectomies due to a genetic mutation may be having feelings of guilt, especially if your child got the gene from you. Of course, there's no blame here. We don't have control of our genetics—neither the genes given to us by our parents or those we pass on to our children.

Jeff, the father of our patient Cara Scharf, had helped take care of Cara's mother as she was dying of metastatic breast cancer in her early forties. Cara was three at the time. Breast cancer was not discussed frequently as Cara grew up, but when she was twenty-two, her father encouraged her to have genetic testing, which showed a BRCA1 mutation. We met Jeff, a practicing obstetrician/gynecologist, when Cara was diagnosed with triple-negative breast cancer at the age of twenty-five. It was found on her first MRI. She was afraid to tell her father about the abnormal MRI, but as soon as she found out the pathology results, she called him. They cried together. From that moment on, Jeff was a constant force in Cara's life, not only supporting her as she worked through the decision of whether to have mastectomies but also staying with her as she underwent her chemotherapy treatments. He even participated in a documentary for our patients and their families (you can see it at https://cancercenter.gwu.edu/profile/patient/cara-scharf).[1] Although he was trained to appear stoic as a physician, he admitted that it had been very emotional to watch everything his daughter went through. He shared tears of joy with her when she had her last chemotherapy session. By encouraging Cara to have genetic testing, Jeff saved his daughter's life. Because she knew her BRCA1 mutation meant she needed to start having imaging at the age of twenty-five, she had a mammogram (which was normal), and six months later, she had the fateful MRI. Without the MRI, she wouldn't have known that she had breast cancer until it was much more advanced.

When Caitlynn Jones was diagnosed with triple-negative right breast cancer at the age of twenty-nine, her mother was right by her side. Her husband and friend often accompanied her to chemotherapy. Her mother had had mastectomies with implants when she was forty-nine, so she was a wonderful support for Caitlynn when she had her own breasts removed. Caitlynn chose to have DIEP reconstructions. As she was interviewed by the anesthesiologists before she began the ten-hour surgery and long recovery, her mother broke down in tears. It was hard to see her child go through something like that, even when she had been through so much of it herself. She admitted that she struggled with the guilt she felt that her daughter had inherited the same BRCA mutation from her. But for Caitlynn, knowing that her mother had gone through mastectomies for breast cancer and was alive and doing well, made her feel completely confident that she, too, was going to beat breast cancer. Caitlynn's confidence helped her mother to provide the support that Caitlynn needed.

Our patient Sylvia was eighty-five years old when she lost her husband and was diagnosed with bilateral breast cancer. It was a difficult double blow to her and her family. When she heard her options for mastectomies, Sylvia was adamant that she wanted full reconstruction. For all of her adult life, she had been five feet tall with extremely large breasts. Her breasts were very important to her. Her children had imagined that she would welcome mastectomies to reduce the size of her breasts, but that was the last thing she wanted. Even though the surgery was longer and the recovery more difficult, she endured it for the sake of feeling as feminine as she always had. Her breasts were always an important part of her sense of attractiveness. For her family, it was an unexpected insight into how their mother felt about her body and how important our physical sense of self can be, even in older age. As with the entire breast cancer journey, open communication is critical. The importance of their mother's breasts to her was an epiphany for her family, but it was also an opportunity to gain more insight into their mother and further support her. This once again emphasizes the importance of listening. Patients *will* tell you what they want and often what they need. The role of a loved one is to listen carefully enough to hear the messages the patient is sending. So sometimes it's necessary to curtail the desire to talk and give advice and to focus on listening. Listening is key to supporting. Even after we've known one another for decades, disease causes us to learn even more about those who are closest to us.

PARTNERS

Cancer has a way of making everything else seem trivial or selfish. It dwarfs the normal, everyday concerns of life. But the truth is, all these things remain extremely important. Perhaps even more important than before.

The impact of breast cancer on one's life partner is profound. Not only do they need to support the person diagnosed with breast cancer, they likely have their own fears, some of which may be about how this difficult time in their partner's life will affect them. Of course, they're terrified by the possibility of losing the person they love and feel enormous sadness for what their partner must go through. However, they may feel guilty for wondering how they will live without the person they love should she lose her battle with breast cancer. If there are young children involved, the fear of raising children alone can weigh heavy. What will life and intimacy be like during and after treatment? These are all legitimate and, in fact, normal emotions. However, they might be mired in guilt for worrying about themselves when their partner is going through a life-threatening illness. They may feel that these emotions are wrong, and their only concern should be their partner. These emotions are normal, and the impact of breast cancer on the life partner/husband/wife/ boyfriend/girlfriend of a woman diagnosed with breast cancer is real and great. The fears and considerations of how breast cancer will affect them shouldn't be causes for guilt.

What advice can we share to help the life partner of a woman with breast cancer? A diagnosis of cancer results in significant emotional distress for both the patient and her partner. There will be challenges and stresses that you could not imagine before the diagnosis. Both the patient and her partner will likely experience sadness, anxiety, anger, even hopelessness. It's not uncommon for the patient going through breast cancer treatment to need extra reassurance that they're still loved. Couples need to be sensitive to the changing emotional needs that come following a diagnosis of cancer. Thoughtfully supporting your loved one is critical, because treatment usually brings physical, psychological, and emotional challenges. However, remember that the caregiver/spouse/partner also needs support. It may be helpful for you as the partner to share your anxieties with a close friend or a support group. However, if the woman undergoing breast cancer treatment senses that you as her partner feel overwhelmed or vulnerable, she may be reticent to share her concerns and fears with you. Nevertheless, you're also going through many difficult changes and need support. Balancing the needs of your loved one with your own needs can be extremely challenging. Take each day one at a time. Some days will be better than others.

The number one most distressing symptom for most cancer survivors is fatigue. It's common during treatment, but can last for weeks, months, and sometimes even years afterward. Hormonal therapy for women with ER-/PR-positive tumors can contribute to exhaustion as well as to some side effects, including hot flashes and joint pain, which can result in sleep disturbances. Her medications may need to be changed or other medications added to help with the hot flashes, and some may cause weight gain.

The impact of breast cancer therapy is profound. There are extensive physical changes from surgery and, if chemotherapy or radiation therapy is part of the treatment, extensive consequences of these often lifesaving treatments. It's critical that you be supportive of the side effects of therapy. When your loved one is fatigued, take over responsibilities to allow them to rest. If they have complications of chemotherapy, be available at a moment's notice. When they want to talk, be there for them. As a caretaker, perhaps one of the most important things is to understand that no matter how much you care and want to help, there are times when your ability to do so is limited. Unfortunately, no matter how devoted you are, you can't fix everything. In those situations, finding the right words or the right nonverbal communication can be extremely helpful, and may be just what's needed.

SEX AFTER BREAST CANCER

After a breast cancer diagnosis, sex may be painful and your libido decreased due to the antihormone treatment or chemotherapy. This, coupled with body image challenges, can impact sexuality. However, it's important to remember that sex and intimacy are not the same. Even if sex is temporarily not feasible, intimacy is never more needed. Thinking creatively about intimacy can be extremely helpful. Communication is extremely important, as are ways of expressing love and closeness through different forms of physical love. Even if a woman doesn't desire intercourse as she goes through treatments, physical touch is important. Holding hands, hugging, and giving massages are only a few examples. Though it's undoubtedly different, it's important to remember that like so much after a cancer diagnosis, sex, too, will return to normal, albeit often a new normal.

Some women will want to continue to have sex during treatment. It can maintain the intimacy in the relationship they crave. In this case, women should discuss this with their oncologists, as some chemotherapy can be secreted in bodily fluids and a condom may be recommended, and oral sex may not be safe for some short period of time after receiving chemotherapy. Some women will need time during and after treatment to heal before resuming sex. Some women have significant issues with the change in their bodies after treatment and may need counseling prior to resuming sex. Every person is different.

During treatment, often a spouse/partner will need to take on many of the tasks previously undertaken by the patient, whether those involve housework, childcare, or other responsibilities. In families with young children, the task of maintaining some semblance of normalcy will often fall on the spouse/partner. However, this is a time that asking for help is important. Perhaps your friends can start a meal train and take on the shared responsibility of delivering meals to your home, or perhaps others can take over dropping off and picking up children from school. Not only will it be helpful to you but it will help your friends find a way to have a positive effect during a trying time in your life. Think of this help as a gift your family and friends want to share with you.

DATING AND BREAST CANCER

The burden of introducing a cancer diagnosis or an increased risk for cancer in the beginning of a relationship is enormous. When do you tell your boyfriend or girlfriend that you have this risk, and that if the relationship continues, it will undoubtedly be impacted by the probability of having cancer or surgery? It's never easy, but it is doable, and the outcome can result in a stronger relationship. How do women with breast cancer date, and when do they broach the topic of breast cancer? Every relationship is different, and every woman and couple approach it differently, but it's comforting to know that many times, this unfathomably difficult task ends positively. But not always.

Rachel was just seventeen when she began to date her now husband, Henry. She shared with him that she was certain she, too, would ultimately have breast cancer. With her mother's diagnosis of breast cancer at the age of thirty-three and maternal aunt's diagnosis at thirty-six, she was absolutely sure. When Henry proposed to Rachel, she was thrilled. But she was also sure that breast cancer would profoundly impact their lives and that Henry might want to reconsider, since breast cancer was a given, and an enormous burden. This was before any genetic mutations had been identified. Henry didn't share Rachel's certainty of breast cancer but assured her that no matter what happened, they would handle everything and anything together and that he was not at all deterred by her family history or her certainty of breast cancer. Rachel was heartened by Henry's promise of unwavering love and commitment to share everything life would bring. And as it turned out, they were both right. Rachel was diagnosed with breast cancer at thirty-seven and Henry was steadfast in his love, as her supportive, ever-present partner.

Dating is full of unknowns already. Adding cancer to the mix can feel like an enormous burden. But sometimes the outcome can reveal that you've found a person who's much stronger and more reliable than you would ever have been able to otherwise know. Sometimes, magical things can happen.

Our patient Melinda, twenty-nine, had been dating Michael for only six months, but she felt that their relationship was very strong. Both of them sensed shortly after they met that they would spend the rest of their lives together. When Melinda was diagnosed with breast cancer and had to leave her job, she lost her health insurance. Michael told her he had wanted to ask her to marry him since they met. They married for love, but they moved the date up and married at city hall the following month so Michael could add Melinda to his health insurance plan. This way, Melinda was able to afford the treatments that she needed for optimal care. A year later, after surgery, chemotherapy, and radiation, Melinda and Michael had the beautiful wedding they had dreamed about.

The fact is, many women in young, strong relationships find that the difficulty of having breast cancer or the burden of a markedly increased risk of breast cancer can actually bring them and their partner closer together. Donna Morgan was diagnosed with triple-negative breast cancer at the age of thirty-two. She was three months into a relationship with her boyfriend, and he had just met her parents. He was there with her every step of the way through surgery and chemotherapy. Since she tested positive for a BRCA1 mutation, she elected to have bilateral mastectomies with implant reconstructions. Her parents were hesitant about her decision— no one in the family had had breast cancer, but ultimately it was found that the mutation came from her father, who had no female family members aside from his mother. In contrast, her boyfriend was immediately supportive and became her strongest advocate. Donna followed her instincts to have the bilateral mastectomies with implant reconstructions, and twenty years later is still thriving. Her boyfriend became her husband, and they're enjoying their lives together raising two children.

The people who will make the best partners—regardless of their age or gender—will rise to the occasion when you're faced with cancer. It's important to remember that facing breast cancer is hard for the patient, their life partner, their family, and their friends. But facing the challenges of breast cancer can bring people closer together.

Dating can also be stressful for single women who were treated for breast cancer or had preventive mastectomies due to an increased risk for breast cancer. When do they tell the person they're dating about their history?

Jennifer is a twenty-nine-year-old BRCA1 patient who, at the age of twenty-six, underwent prophylactic mastectomies with beautiful reconstructions. Shortly after she began to date her now husband, Michael, she realized that the relationship was becoming more serious and she had to share with him that she had undergone bilateral prophylactic mastectomies. She began the conversation with "I have something very important I need to tell you . . ." He had no idea what to expect. When she shared her situation and the surgery she'd had, he was so relieved and unfazed. The increased risk of breast cancer and potentially other cancers, as well as the prophylactic mastectomies, never impacted his love for or commitment to Jennifer. They're now married and have two beautiful children.

When Christy's friend Laurie met Brant, she knew there was an immediate connection. On their first date, she told him about her breast cancer and all the treatments she endured. She also told him about how her father had died from breast cancer. She didn't want to get involved in a relationship without full disclosure. She had already gone through a difficult breakup just as she completed all her cancer treatments when she was thirty-five. But she could tell that Brant was different, and it was not long before she knew that if she ever faced breast cancer again, he would be there for her. A year after they were married, she was again diagnosed with breast cancer. He was, and still is, at her side.

COMMUNITY SUPPORT

As essential as loved ones are in times like these, you may find power, companionship, connection, and inspiration by seeking out a broader community. Even with supportive loved ones who are there for you, you may need the understanding of those facing similar challenges. Only those in similar situations can fully understand what you're going through.

You need not limit yourself to your own circle of loved ones to find people who have shared your experience. So many wonderful support communities for cancer have grown out of the prevalence of this disease, where you can readily find warm, loving people who understand what you're going through—your fear of the procedures, your worries about their impact on your relationships, your adjustments to the treatments, your recovery efforts, even starting life again on the other side of remission. As the global organization Cancer Support Community rightly says, "Community Is Stronger Than Cancer."[2]

Many hospitals have support groups for people undergoing cancer therapy as well as survivorship support groups. These may be for women with breast cancer or may be directed at specific people—whether it's support groups for young women with breast cancer, older women with breast cancer, or those with mutations that substantially increase their risk of breast cancer. There are support groups out there for you, and you may find them exceedingly helpful.

Chemotherapy and hormone therapy can have significant side effects, including emotional and mood issues. The fear of recurrence is not uncommon for women who have completed treatment for breast cancer. It's important to know that most women who have a supportive, loving caregiver get through treatment better than those who are isolated. Research has shown that chronic loneliness worsens outcomes from breast cancer treatment. Having strong social ties, both with family as well as friends and community, is critical, and those who don't have this important support have a higher risk of recurrence and poorer survival.[3]

COLLEAGUES AT WORK

So many of us are faced with a colleague at work who has been diagnosed with breast cancer. Remember, some women can't wait to get back to work and to as much normalcy as possible. Some women can barely get through the day for both physical and emotional reasons, so work is out of the question. Everyone will need additional time off for doctor's appointments and procedures. Here are some specific suggestions for supporting your coworker through her breast cancer journey:

- Ask her if she wants others to know about her diagnosis and whether she'd like you to help her share the news, especially if you're her manager.
- If you're her manager, discuss sick leave and financial options with as much flexibility and compassion as possible. Kindness in a time of need is forever remembered.
- Be flexible with time off for doctor's appointments, tests, and treatment.
- Before she returns to work, discuss any limitations that may apply. Be aware that how she feels may change from day to day or week to week. Arrange for someone to help out if the workload gets to be too much.
- Be yourself and maintain your relationship, always remembering to let her know you care and understand that these are challenging times.

- Include her in social events. She may not be able to sustain a workday, but sometimes she might greatly appreciate being included in outside activities.
- Ask her what she can and cannot do.

DO NOT

- Avoid her.
- Ask inappropriate or prying questions. It's not reasonable to ask why she got cancer, whether she has a family history of it, or if she had a lifestyle that increased the risk of cancer, like smoking or alcohol intake. It's not appropriate.
- Make assumptions about what she can and cannot do. Ask her.

SILVER LININGS

Hard as it is to imagine, there can be silver linings during breast cancer treatment. Our patients often describe a greater appreciation for the gifts of life: the smiles of their children, the kindness of friends and family, the love of their partners.

Of course, any woman undergoing breast cancer treatment has to come to terms with changes to her body, deal with the fear of death, and become "the cancer patient." The journey can be difficult, and there can be unexpected complications. However, at the end of treatment, life will return to normal, only it will be a "new normal." The invincibility that some feel before being diagnosed with breast cancer won't be the same, and the journey will bring a challenging chapter to your life. However, you will overcome it and be assured that you will laugh again, enjoy life again, and find some new normal that you will be able to live with.

You may also find that the kindness of others is magnified in times of need and that loving acts of kindness come from many unexpected places. Rachel was diagnosed with breast cancer two months before her eldest daughter's bat mitzvah. So many friends and acquaintances helped her with every aspect of planning that very special day in her and her family's life. Rachel was so deeply touched by their kindness and generosity. Her daughter's bat mitzvah was filled with joy, laughter, and gratitude.

Rachel also felt profound gratitude during her chemotherapy. Before her diagnosis of breast cancer, life moved at breakneck speed, with the chaotic needs of a hectic young family with three school-age children, two busy clinical practices, exciting groundbreaking research, and seemingly endless responsibilities pulling in so many directions. After the diagnosis, Rachel gained a greater appreciation of the laughter of her children and the love of her husband in ways that weren't possible before her diagnosis. While many women choose to do their chemotherapy toward the end of the week so they have the weekend to recover, Rachel did her treatments in the beginning of the week so she could feel well enough on the weekend to enjoy time with her family. She also learned to take time off from work when she needed it. Being a workaholic, this was new to her, and something she welcomed during her surgery and chemotherapy.

Christy looks back at the time she had off work while she recovered from surgery with fond memories. Her husband, Dave, was a rock as she made the decision to have mastectomies, and provided the support she needed after the surgery. Not having to worry about treatments for cancer because she had had preventive mastectomies meant she only had to focus on her recovery. The very basics of life can be exhausting in those first weeks after surgery. Taking naps was essential, and Christy now recommends that her patients listen to their bodies and rest as much as possible. When her friend Laurie came to visit the first week after surgery, all they did was watch movies and play computer games. To this day, Christy treasures those memories. Having family and loved ones nearby and knowing that they were there for her during those first few weeks resulted in a quicker and easier recovery for Christy.

Experts agree that gratitude from finding the good in a sea of overwhelming challenges results in a more resilient and tolerable response to hardships. While you're undergoing the physical challenges of breast cancer treatments and recovery, it can be hard to see the silver linings. The whole world can feel as if it's in a fog. When you reconnect with it, you may experience it in a different way than before. Loved ones are the resource for helping you through a time that can have so many unnerving and disorienting moments. Whether they're driving you to an appointment, holding your hand, or texting to make sure you're okay, those supporting you can ensure that you stay in touch with the great healing powers of gratitude, happiness, and love.

CHAPTER 11

The Future

W e've stood on the shoulders of giants with innumerable scientific and clinical discoveries to achieve an incredible feat: decreasing the death rate from breast cancer by more than 40 percent.

Two decades ago, we didn't have targeted therapy, where we administer drugs to wipe out specific cancer cells while sparing the normal cells. We now offer estrogen-blocking drugs to those whose breast cancers have estrogen receptors, and Herceptin to those who have HER2-neu receptors. We've moved into the realm of personalized precision medicine, where we treat breast cancers based on genetics. This has dramatically improved our ability to assess who will respond best to what kind of chemotherapy in how many doses.

These are only some of the reasons we've seen remarkable declines in the death rate from breast cancer. And the future stands before us like a bright, shining beacon, because the discoveries in development now are even more exciting.

Extraordinary strides in risk-based screening for breast cancer have been critical in impacting the decrease in breast cancer deaths. When Rachel began in the field of breast imaging, breast cancer screening involved only mammography, which had itself reduced the death rate from breast cancer by 20 percent.[1] During the first few decades of breast imaging, we were taught *not* to use ultrasound to screen for breast cancer. Now we know that some women should have screening with ultrasound, either handheld or automated, in addition to their annual screening mammogram, every year! We've learned that essential screening—a term used by Andrea Wolf, former CEO of the Brem Foundation, to describe risk-based screening that includes ultrasound, MRI, or other modalities as needed based on the individual woman's needs (previously called adjunct screening)—allows for the detection of 25 percent more cancers. In women with dense breasts, ultrasound finds cancers that hide in tissue that shows up white on mammography. It's essential to search for these hidden killer cancers to improve breast cancer outcomes for those women.

Over the years, we've modified our use of MRI as new data has supported its expanded use in screening women who are at substantially increased risk of breast cancers, such as those with BRCA mutations. In fact, the American Cancer Society now recommends annual MRI screening for every woman with a 20 percent or greater lifetime risk of breast cancer, and consideration of an annual MRI in those with a 15 to 20 percent lifetime risk. And in Pennsylvania, legislation requires insurance coverage of MRI screening for women with extremely dense breasts. MRIs can find cancers not seen with any other imaging. This allows us to detect more early, curable breast cancers.

We've traversed a monumental change in information and clinical practice in a remarkably short period of time! We now are committed to risk-based screening to optimize the ability to detect early, curable breast cancer.

Timeline of Medical Advances for Breast Cancer

1882: First radical mastectomy for breast cancer. The procedure was performed by Johns Hopkins Hospital surgeon William Stewart Halsted.[2] It remained the standard treatment into the twentieth century.

1937: Radiation therapy used to spare the breast. Needles containing radium were inserted into the breast near the lymph nodes after the tumor was removed.[3]

1974: Chemotherapy approved by the FDA for breast cancer treatment. After the sulfuric mustard gas used in World War I affected the lymph nodes and bone marrow of soldiers, Pfizer developed doxorubicin (Adriamycin) and got FDA approval for its use for breast cancer treatment.[4]

1978: Tamoxifen approved by the FDA for breast cancer treatment. Tamoxifen was the first of a new class of drugs known as selective estrogen receptor modulators (SERMs).[5] Approved for primary prevention in 1999, it reduced the incidence of the disease by about 30 percent.[6]

1980s: Lumpectomy over radical mastectomy. A study by University of Pittsburgh surgeon Bernard Fisher made the less-invasive breast conservation surgery (lumpectomy) with radiation therapy more popular when it was shown to have the same survival rate as radical mastectomy.[7]

1994: BRCA1 gene discovered. Dr. Mary-Claire King discovered the location and role of the BRCA1 gene in hereditary breast and ovarian cancers.[8]

2000s: Preventive mastectomies for BRCA mutations. New studies investigated the value of preventive mastectomies for BRCA-positive patients.[9]

2001: Breast cancer seen as many diseases. Charles Perou, MD, reclassified breast cancer as a collection of diseases, which are based on different patterns of genes.[10]

2007: Additional screening for BRCA mutations. The American Cancer Society recommends high-risk women receive regular screening with MRI.[11]

2009: Preventive surgery for high-risk carriers. Removal of the breasts, ovaries, and fallopian tubes is proven to reduce the risk of breast cancer in those with BRCA gene mutations.[12]

2018: New guidelines for chemotherapy use. New studies show that 70 percent of women with early-stage breast cancer do not need chemotherapy, allowing for better definition of which breast cancer patients benefit from the treatment.[13]

We've made incredible strides in our understanding of breast cancer and its causes, as well as in our protocols for treatment and our technology. We live in very exciting times; we're integrating these novel developing technologies into our clinical practices at a rate that has never been possible before. With so much on the horizon, let's review some of the recent and anticipated developments in breast cancer screening, diagnosis, and treatment. Of course, these are but a few.

ADVANCES IN PERSONALIZED MEDICINE

Personalized medicine is often called precision medicine because it allows us to precisely calibrate a treatment to the individual. When this approach is applied to cancer treatment, it can target cancerous cells more accurately and leave healthy cells alone as much as possible.[14]

Pharmacogenomics

We now know so much more about how any given treatment or medication will interact with the genes you've inherited. Because of genetic differences, a drug that's safe and effective for one woman may be damaging or completely ineffective for another. The same dose can create no noticeable side effects or intolerable side effects, depending on the person.

Testing how an individual's genes respond to drugs or treatments with pharmacogenomics may be able to improve therapy. We may find the appropriate medications, treatments, and doses for your individual genetic profile. As a result, you can undergo the very necessary treatments for cancer with more confidence that they will work and be safe for you.

Many people process one particular drug faster than average. It's important to know if that's the case for you, since it means the drug will move through your system very quickly. Depending on the situation, you may need to take a higher or more frequent dose for the drug to be effective. If you tend to process a certain drug more slowly, it will linger in your bloodstream longer. That could be why you experience more side effects than others. When you can identify the genetic basis for this reaction with pharmacogenomics, your doctor will know to give you a lower dose of that medication.[15] These distinctive reactions are true not just for drugs but for medical treatments, recovery times, supplemental aids, and many other elements in your overall plan. The beauty of precision medicine is that it can offer your doctor powerful insights into how they can best optimize your treatment for you.

Tailoring treatments to the individual has brought about a dramatic change in medicine. Two decades ago, we could not predict who would or would not benefit from chemotherapy. When Rachel was diagnosed with breast cancer, the standard protocol followed was chemotherapy in all women with a one-centimeter (approximately half an inch) or larger tumor. We knew that some women benefited from this therapy and some did not. However, we could not yet predict who would and who would not. Now we can.

In those days, we didn't yet have genomic tests like Oncotype DX or MammaPrint that can tell you how likely it is that your breast cancer will recur or spread. Today, that's an important part of our testing. These great strides in bench-to-bedside research have already become part of our everyday patient care, with an extraordinary impact on women's health.

ADVANCES IN SCREENING
Artificial Intelligence Applications

Harnessing the power of artificial intelligence (AI) will undoubtedly ensure faster, earlier detection of breast cancer and save more lives. AI is the ability of a computer or a robot controlled by a computer to do tasks that are usually done by humans that require the ability to make a decision. Artificial intelligence is increasingly being used all around us. Businesses use AI to make strategic decisions; self-driving vehicles use AI to make decisions on the road. Apple's Siri, Google Now, Amazon's Alexa, and Microsoft's Cortana are digital assistants that use AI to help users perform tasks from checking their schedules and searching for something on the web to sending commands to another app. These digital assistants learn from every choice you make and make their next suggestions based on what you've chosen in the past. AI is also increasingly being used in medicine and in particular in the diagnosis of breast cancer.

The success rate of mammography is dramatically improved when screening has the benefit of augmentation with AI. Mammography is particularly well suited for AI, since it's searching for only one thing: breast cancer. AI scans mammograms for the features of breast cancer. This is exciting, since research has demonstrated that even the best breast imagers don't see all cancers on mammograms. As a result, radiologists are able to identify more cancers in less time—and computers never get tired like people do. Studies have also shown that when general radiologists use AI for mammography, they can be as accurate and skilled as a subspecialized breast imager in finding cancers on mammograms, and that less experienced radiologists perform as well as very experienced radiologists when they use AI in their interpretation. In Europe, many countries require that a mammogram be interpreted by two radiologists, but the medical profession has experienced shortages in recent years, making it increasingly challenging for second radiologists to be available. Researchers have determined that when used by one interpreting radiologist, AI works at least as well as a second radiologist.[16]

Adding AI can have profound implications on how accurately mammograms can be interpreted and how many mammograms can be interpreted to save more lives. A recent study has demonstrated that the use of Transpara Breast Care AI can reduce the radiologists' work by 62 percent,[17] making radiologists available to interpret many more lifesaving mammograms around the globe. It opens the door to very exciting possibilities, and it's already in use today.

AI AND MAMMOGRAPHY

As many as 40 percent of breast cancers are not visible with mammography in women with dense breasts due to the masking effect of the white breast tissue on mammography. This is an expected limitation of mammography. However, we can improve this as well as the limitation of human performance where radiologists can be less experienced, tired, or not specialized in breast imaging. These limitations can be improved and indeed erased by the groundbreaking application of artificial intelligence to mammography.

The FDA has cleared several AI products for mammography, and these are now increasingly being used clinically. AI will allow radiologists to diagnose breast cancer cases earlier, at more curable stages. AI alone, without a radiologist, isn't cleared by the FDA yet, but it may well be in the future, since AI alone works nearly as well as a subspecialized radiologist and, with further development, may work as well as (or perhaps even better than) a radiologist.

AI FOR BREAST ULTRASOUND AND BREAST MRI

Another recent development is AI for breast ultrasound. Some AI products for breast ultrasound are already available clinically, and these not only help identify cancers but can help analyze lesions that are found to better assess whether they're cancer. Several groups of researchers and companies are working to further develop and improve AI for breast ultrasound.

Similarly, research into the use of MRI to identify and characterize abnormal lesions is ongoing and will soon be introduced into clinical practice.

RACIAL AND ECONOMIC EQUITY

One incredibly exciting possibility AI can offer is a way to rebalance the racial disparity that exists in breast cancer. Studies have shown that women from underserved communities in the US who receive breast cancer care at Centers of Excellence have far improved survival rates than those who get care in their home communities.[18] Women of color have a 40 percent higher death rate from breast cancer than white women, in part due to the economic disparity in communities of color.[19] AI can move toward helping women receiving care at the Centers of Excellence level even when they aren't being cared for in one. It should have a profound impact on the unacceptable difference in breast cancer care in underserved communities. There is a recent preliminary report suggesting bias in the development of AI regarding underrepresented minorities. We must be certain to optimize AI to impact healthcare disparities by utilizing it for the optimal interpretation of breast imaging studies in underrepresented minorities, and to make sure that adequate numbers of underrepresented women are included in the development of AI.

Globally, AI may have an even greater impact. In lower-income countries, there's virtually no breast cancer screening, even though breast cancer is the most common cancer among women worldwide. In these countries, the death rate from breast cancer nearly parallels the incidence of the disease. The greatest reason there's little or no breast cancer screening is the unavailability of doctors to interpret mammograms. Imagine how many lives could be saved if there were screening programs where mammography machines were placed in rural areas and the mammograms evaluated with AI alone. More than 95 percent of the mammograms will be appropriately identified as negative without ever being read by a radiologist.[20] The less than 5 percent of women whose mammograms were not flagged as negative will then go to centralized diagnostic centers for ongoing evaluation. This one change could have an unimaginable positive impact on the death rate from breast cancer around the globe.

MRI Innovations

Our patients often ask, "If MRI is the most sensitive test for finding breast cancer, why don't we use that instead of mammography or ultrasound?"

First, an MRI is a very expensive examination that requires the intravenous injection of a contrast dye (often gadolinium, a heavy metal) to better visualize cancers in the image. Studies have shown that with multiple MRIs, gadolinium can accumulate in the brain.[21] Although we believe it has no detrimental effect, it would be better to obtain the information without the use of contrast. Fortunately, there are two new types of MRI, one that doesn't require contrast and one that allows for greater availability of the MRIs that are currently available.

- **Diffusion-weighted MRI:** This type of MRI study has the potential to image breast cancer without contrast dye (gadolinium). To date, studies have demonstrated its potential, but additional technical developments are required to image small cancers, as well as to standardize the examination to make it available in clinical practice.
- **Abbreviated MRI:** Increasingly, abbreviated MRIs are being used to screen high-risk women. Although it still requires

the injection of contrast dye, the examination is much shorter, since fewer images are required. The shorter time in the machine not only makes it more comfortable for women but also makes the machine more available for additional exams. Currently, most medical insurance doesn't cover abbreviated breast MRIs. Several institutions have created relatively low-cost abbreviated breast MRI programs and encouraged woman at increased risk to pay for the screening out of pocket. Once hospitals and insurance companies come to recognize how many more women can be imaged with abbreviated MRI, the hope is that they will cover these lifesaving examinations.

Ultrasound Tomography

A very exciting technology developed for precision medicine in recent years is SoftVue 3D ultrasound tomography by Delphinus, which was recently FDA approved.[22] It uses the same type of safe ultrasound waves used to image fetuses in the womb, but the transducer (the device that actually images) has been developed to better understand and inform about the tissue characteristics. As such, not only does SoftVue detect more cancers, it also helps determine which findings are cancer and which are not more accurately, reducing the number of biopsies necessary after screening.

Preliminary research has shown that SoftVue has many other exciting possibilities. Currently, in neoadjuvant treatment, several courses of chemotherapy are needed before it can be determined if a woman is responding to the chemotherapy or if she isn't and the specific drugs being used should be changed. A small study determined that SoftVue can show this very early in neoadjuvant treatment, meaning adjustments to the chemotherapy drugs can be made earlier as well. Additionally, a preliminary study demonstrated that the use of SoftVue can more accurately determine a woman's breast cancer risk,[23] though more research is needed to confirm this finding.

Breast density is a critical factor in determining a woman's breast cancer risk. It's increasingly being used in calculating a woman's risk profile. Until now, we've only been able to determine a woman's breast density with mammography, which uses radiation—something we want to avoid whenever possible and especially in younger women, whose breasts are more sensitive to radiation than those of older women. SoftVue can help us do just that, as it can determine a woman's breast density without ionizing radiation. This new technology is a game changer. More studies are needed to evaluate its role in clinical practice, but this FDA-approved device will soon be available clinically.

ADVANCES IN DIAGNOSIS

Liquid Biopsies

Normally, a definitive diagnosis of breast cancer requires a tissue sample. The trouble is that by the time a cancer is large enough to see on imaging or feel in a physical examination, it has been there for some time, maybe even years. A very small breast cancer that measures half a centimeter (less than a quarter of an inch) is already composed of *ten million cancer cells*. Some of these cancer cells circulate in the blood long before a mass is visible or can be felt. In fact, the number of circulating cancer cells can be indicative of the likelihood of developing metastases or how well you will do. Analyzing blood and other bodily fluids for cancer cells or cancer DNA is called liquid biopsy.

The FDA has approved liquid biopsy for patients with metastatic breast, colon, or prostate cancers. This test can be done serially and help predict the effectiveness of treatment as well as prognosis. Researchers have found that women with cancer cells in their blood are *twice as likely* to die of their disease as women who do not.[24] This is because metastatic disease, in part, depends on cancer cells spreading from the original site of the tumor to other parts of the body. However, getting repeat blood samples and evaluating them for these cells or DNA during treatment can help doctors modify treatment to make it as effective as possible. In some women with metastatic disease, serial liquid biopsies may be helpful to determine the efficacy of their care. While liquid biopsies have shown promising results, they aren't yet considered standard of care in the management of patients. Ask your physician whether there's a potential role for sequential liquid biopsies in your treatment (at this point, the answer is likely "not yet").

Although it's a remarkable development, there are some challenges. One challenge is that a patient may be found to have cancer cells or cancer DNA in their liquid biopsy but not actually have cancer. This is called a false positive and, as you can imagine, is problematic. Imagine being told you have tumor DNA in your blood only to find out after extensive testing that you do not, in fact, have cancer. Currently, research is investigating combining DNA findings with other findings such as protein markers to make the test more accurate.

Even with their limitations, liquid biopsies are one of the most exciting advances in breast cancer and, indeed, many other cancers. It's increasingly being integrated into clinical practice and will likely be a critical way to diagnose the earliest, most curable breast cancers as well as how effective ongoing cancer treatments.[25]

ADVANCES IN SURGERY

Lymphatic Reconstruction

Surgery to remove the axillary lymph nodes is necessary if more than two lymph node test positive for cancer. Afterward, the inner arm will be numb or experience tingling. This can be temporary, but if there's swelling of the arm later after the surgery, a condition known as lymphedema, it's more concerning. As many as 20 to 40 percent of women experience lymphedema after lymph node removal.[26] We recommend wearing a compression sleeve to avoid it, but specialized plastic surgeons have developed a better alternative. They offer immediate lymphatic reconstruction to patients who need axillary lymph node dissection. First, they inject a dye into the inner upper arm and use a microscope to observe the lymphatics draining from the arm. In this remarkable procedure, they then do microscopic surgery to attach the lymphatics to blood vessels so the fluid can drain.

Ultimately, this surgical procedure may significantly reduce the rate of lymphedema and improve women's quality of life. Already, some limited studies have shown a significantly reduced rate, as low as 3 to 4 percent.[27] Others have shown rates from 4 to 12 percent.[28]

Radiation, Not Surgery

Long-term data shows that patients with one or two positive sentinel lymph nodes don't need complete axillary lymph node dissections as long as they're having radiation to the breast. The radiation treats the lymph nodes at the same time. Patients have an equal survival and recurrence rate whether their lymph nodes are removed or not.

Emerging data indicates that patients being treated with chemotherapy might also be able to avoid a dissection, as long as there's no evidence of tumor cells after the primary cancer surgery. Pending studies are evaluating whether radiation can replace axillary lymph node dissection for patients who still have residual cancer in their lymph node(s) after chemotherapy.[29]

Nipple Sensation Preserved

Quality of life is an important consideration in breast cancer treatment, and no woman is happy about the loss of sensation in her nipples, even if the surgery was essential. Until recently, we've had very few options to address this, and the difficult reality has been that sensation is lost in nipple-sparing mastectomies. But now, advanced surgical techniques in preserving sensation in the hands after nerve repair are finally giving women hope.[30]

Using microsurgery, plastic surgeons are learning how to reconnect the sensory nerves in the chest that are cut during the mastectomy. This may be performed with or without a nerve graft. The procedure requires specialized training and has yet to gain widespread adoption, so few plastic surgeons currently offer it, but its appeal is undisputable. Although only specially trained plastic surgeons offer this procedure at the time of this writing, many more will be trained by the time this book is published. This website continues to be updated with providers trained in performing nerve reconstruction: resensation.com.

We continue to be honest and up front with our patients that sensation cannot be guaranteed, but we're working hard to make it possible. It can take months to years to know if sensation will be restored, as nerves regenerate at a rate of one to two millimeters per day. Even if there's a successful nerve identification and repair, sensation isn't guaranteed, but there is hope for the future.[31]

Endocrine Therapy

Ductal carcinoma in situ (DCIS) is a cancer in the milk ducts of the breast. It doesn't have the ability to spread and is always considered stage 0. About 75 percent of DCIS will not progress to an invasive carcinoma, so most patients won't need surgery or radiation.[32] But since we don't know which 25 percent of patients might safely avoid treatment, surgery and radiation are recommended for all patients. In severe cases, a mastectomy might be recommended. It's clear that most patients are overtreated for DCIS, but without being able to predict whose disease will progress, we prefer to avoid the risk.

A better solution may be in development. A clinical trial for treating low-risk DCIS is underway called the COMET (Comparison of Operative versus Monitoring and Endocrine Therapy) trial. This trial compares patients who have had surgery to those who have been surveilled with mammograms every six months for five years. The surveillance patients have the option of taking hormone therapy to reduce their risk. This is a "wait and see" approach that isn't considered standard of care at this time.[33]

Another study, known as the PREvent Ductal Carcinoma In Situ Overtreatment Now (PRECISION) initiative, aims to learn more about why DCIS turns into invasive breast cancer in some women but not in others. The goal is to determine which patients with DCIS are not at risk for developing invasive breast cancer and can avoid treatment.[34]

One-Stop Breast Cancer Treatment

We've become expert at diagnosing ever smaller cancers. Biopsies of breast abnormalities should be minimally invasive procedures using a needle instead of a knife, and now we're beginning to develop methods to treat breast cancers minimally invasively by freezing or with heat, so that in the future surgery may not be necessary. We're moving into an era when we can even give radiation therapy at the time of breast surgery, in the operating room. What has been missing is the ability to determine if the margins of excised breast cancer are clear (or negative) of any residual tissue on the margin. That's called margin assessment. We now can improve our accuracy with a device called MarginProbe, which allows determination of negative margins with greater accuracy. With all these pieces in place and with continued development of each part of this process, we can foresee a time in the not-too-distant future when a woman can be diagnosed and treated for her breast cancer at the same time, or with one stop. This is very exciting, as it would minimize the trauma of breast cancer treatment.

Preimplantation Genetic Diagnosis (PGD)
If you have a mutation or some other inherited gene associated with increased risk of breast cancer or other cancers, it's natural to be concerned about passing the mutation along to your biological children. There's a 50 percent chance that any child you have will inherit the mutation if you or your partner carry the gene. Some women of childbearing age are now choosing to use preimplantation genetic diagnosis (PGD) to ensure they won't pass a mutation on to their children. PGD has been used for some time to prevent children from inheriting diseases such as cystic fibrosis, muscular dystrophy, and Huntington's disease. Now some parents use PGD to avoid passing cancer genes to their children.

With PGD, a woman undergoes in vitro fertilization (IVF). A few days after her eggs are harvested and fertilized, they're tested for the abnormal gene. Only those fertilized eggs without the gene are implanted in the woman's uterus or stored for future use. In that way, a woman or a couple can ensure that their biological children will not carry the deleterious gene that she or her partner carries.

There are issues with PGD. It's expensive, time-consuming,

and requires numerous medical procedures. In addition, BRCA and other genetic mutations for breast cancer are not diseases but rather indicators of high risk for a disease. Nevertheless, consideration of PGD for those with a cancer gene mutation is reasonable, possible, and increasingly being used.

CONCLUSION

Until not a single woman dies of breast cancer, we will continue to work tirelessly and creatively to find new and emerging technologies to fight the ongoing battle of breast cancer. The good news is that the death rate from breast cancer has markedly decreased over the past two decades. We're fortunate to live in these times during which enormous strides have been made, and many more will undoubtedly follow with profound impact.

Some of these new technologies will benefit us soon. Many more will be discovered in the coming years. We haven't been able to cover all the potential diagnostic and therapeutic developments in this book, but many exciting, novel, and unimaginable advances, such as genomic-based screening and breast cancer vaccines, are coming our way. We didn't even begin to discuss the rapidly changing field of chemotherapy, where more effective and targeted treatments are constantly being introduced along with immunotherapy. As you go through your diagnosis and are deciding which path to pursue, be sure to ask your medical oncologist about clinical trials you might be eligible for. Not only could it benefit you, it might also be part of the clues needed to improve the care for future breast cancer patients. There are so many clinical trials available, so be certain your medical oncologist is familiar with current trials that may help with your treatment. Every clinical trial has different criteria for who can participate, based on what is being studied, so if a study is evaluating new drugs for cancers that are estrogen-receptor-positive (ER-positive) and you don't have estrogen receptors on your particular cancer, you won't qualify. Additionally, specific clinical trials will only be available at a handful of cancer centers, not widely available, so you will need to seek advice about which clinical trials you qualify for, whether you choose to participate, and at what centers those trials are available. It's a lot to research and consider. However, it's critical that clinical trials be part of your care considerations after a diagnosis or recurrence of breast cancer.

Acknowledgments

I wrote this book in memory of my mother, Nancy Brown, and in honor of my best friend, Laurie Turney. They are the reason I decided to specialize in caring for breast cancer patients and those at increased risk for it, and a large part of why I was inspired to write this book. My patients, many of whom are included in the stories you've read throughout the book, are the other main inspiration. When I think about how thankful they all have been for the care they received, I realize this book is for all women who are considering having mastectomies and struggling with the decision.

I've felt incredibly fortunate to work with Rachel for the past twenty-two years; radiologists and surgeons don't always have the bond that we have, and we're lucky to share the same goals of taking great care of patients and offering advice when requested. We have an incredible team of dedicated radiologists and surgeons, all specializing in breast cancer. I always wanted to write a book with Rachel, and when the pandemic started it seemed to provide the opportunity. We both knew the time was right when Gail Ross, literary agent extraordinaire, agreed to take on our proposal. It didn't take long for us to realize that we needed to write a book to help women who were considering the option of mastectomies, either for a diagnosis of breast cancer or for increased risk of it.

Gail guided us and came up with the appropriate title *No Longer Radical*. When Leah Miller accepted our proposal, we knew it was going to be a perfect fit. We couldn't have hoped for a better team. My wish is that our book will help many women in the future as they decide what's best for them, and to know that having mastectomies truly is not radical.

I'm so appreciative of my colleagues Anita McSwain and Joanne Lenert. Anita took amazing care of my mother, and then took care of me. That's a lot of pressure on a colleague, but she handled it with grace and compassion. Joanne gave me beautiful reconstructions, just as she has done these past twenty-two years for all our mutual patients. She is retiring and leaving an empty spot in my professional heart. But more important, I'm thankful for my family. I'm fortunate to have a great relationship with my siblings and their children, who rallied together when our mother was dying of breast cancer and supported me when I had my surgery, and are now excited about this book. Most important, I could never have had preventive mastectomies without the support of my amazing husband, Dave, who was also my cheerleader. every step of the way for this book. My children Ashley, Ellie, and Nick are my ultimate inspiration; every single day with them is a gift.

—Christy Teal

The decisions that face women with breast cancer and those at increased risk of breast cancer are so complex and monumental that they can be overwhelming. We chose to share our expertise and personal experiences as breast cancer doctors and patients to help these women during this journey.

There are so many who must be thanked and without whom this book would never have happened. The commitment and resolve shown by my partner in writing this book, Christy Teal, were steadfast. I'm always amazed by Christy's insightfulness, brilliance, and kindness. I'm grateful every day that she's my colleague and, even more, my friend. Our editor at Simon Element, Leah Miller, "got it" from day one. She understood the need and the passion. Our literary agent, Gail Ross, not only understood the importance but came up with the title of this book. Thank you for being extraordinary partners.

There are so many who helped to instill my passion to ameliorate the pain and difficulties of breast cancer. Ironically, I feel immeasurable gratitude for the good breast cancer has brought to my life, including purpose and focus. My gratitude for the Brem Foundation—a nonprofit founded nearly two decades ago by a group of committed and wonderful friends and patients and dedicated to education, access, and advocacy focused on early detection—is endless. Thank you to Sue Apple and Cheryl Skillin, cofounders of the Brem Foundation, for your wisdom, love, and commitment. I also had the extraordinary opportunity to work closely with my daughter, Andrea Brem Wolf, during her tenure as the CEO of the Brem Foundation.

To my family, without whose support, love, and commitment nothing is possible. First and foremost, to the love of my life, my husband, Henry, who is always there for me and with me. He is prouder of my accomplishments than I am and always sees the good in everyone. Thank you for your incredible insight and your contributions to improving this book. Breast cancer has been far too pervasive a part of us, and yet you never stopped seeing the positives in everything. To my three extraordinary daughters, Andrea Wolf, Alisa Rosenberg, and Sarah Sunshine, whose love, inspiration, and fortitude are endless. My pride for you is immeasurable. You are impacted by breast cancer in ways that others cannot understand and take it all in stride, sometimes through unimaginable challenges. The love, support, and sheer happiness that you bring are never-ending gifts. To my sons-in-law, Ariel Wolf, Jacob Rosenberg, and Joel Sunshine, your ever-present love and kindness are so appreciated. To my ten spectacular grandchildren who shower us with joy and pride every day, you are gifts that never stop giving. I can only hope that your future is one in which breast cancer is known only from history.

Finally, to all the people who will benefit from this book: I understand the difficulties you're going through and sincerely hope that this book brings new perspective, information, and help at a time when they're most needed.

—Rachel Brem

Notes

CHAPTER 1: ARE MASTECTOMIES RIGHT FOR YOU?

1. Hali Hartman, Jie Zhao, and Sujuan Ba, "International Szent-Györgyi Prize for Progress in Cancer Research: Basic and Translational Research Recognition," *Chinese Journal of Cancer* 36 (2017): 92, www.ncbi.nlm.nih.gov/pmc /articles/PMC5697018/.
2. Caroline Helwick, "Dr. Mary-Claire King Proposes Population Screening in All Young Women for *BRCA* Mutations," *ASCO Post*, February 10, 2015, www .ascopost.com/issues/february-10-2015/dr-mary-claire-king -proposes-population-screening-in-all-young-women-for -brca-mutations/.
3. "BRCA Exchange Aggregates Data on Thousands of BRCA Variants to Inform Understanding of Cancer Risk," National Institutes of Health, January 9, 2019, www.nih.gov /news-events/news-releases/brca-exchange-aggregates-data -thousands-brca-variants-inform-understanding-cancer-risk.
4. Cindy Rich, "When a Breast Cancer Surgeon Undergoes a Double Mastectomy," *Washingtonian*, July 5, 2011, www .washingtonian.com/2011/07/05/when-a-breast-cancer -surgeons-mother-undergoes-a-double-mastectomy.
5. Katie Kindelan and Emily O'Donnell, "Confronting a

Family History of Breast Cancer, a Surgeon Makes a Radical Decision," ABC News, June 1, 2011, www .abcnews.go.com/Health/breast-cancer-surgeon-makes -radical-decision-knife/story?id=13731902.

CHAPTER 2: HIGH-RISK SCREENING

1. Carol E. DeSantis et al., "Breast Cancer Statistics, 2019," *CA: A Cancer Journal for Clinicians* 69, no. 6 (November/ December 2019): 438–51, https://acsjournals.onlinelibrary .wiley.com/doi/full/10.3322/caac.21583.

2. "Breast Cancer: Statistics," Cancer.net, January 2022, www.cancer.net/cancer-types/breast-cancer/statistics.

3. Jennifer A. Harvey and Viktor E. Bovbjerg, "Quantitative Assessment of Mammographic Breast Density: Relationship with Breast Cancer Risk," *Radiology* 230, no. 1 (January 2004): 29–41, https://pubs.rsna.org/doi/abs/10.1148 /radiol.2301020870.

4. Etta D. Pisano et al., "Diagnostic Performance of Digital versus Film Mammography for Breast-Cancer Screening," *New England Journal of Medicine* 353, no. 17 (October 2005): 1773–83, https://www.nejm.org/doi/pdf/10.1056 /NEJMoa052911.

5. Rachel F. Brem et al., "Assessing Improvement in Detection of Breast Cancer with Three-Dimensional Automated Breast US in Women with Dense Breast Tissue: The SomoInsight Study," *Radiology* 274, no. 3 (March 2015): 663–73, https://pubmed.ncbi.nlm.nih.gov/25329763/.

6. Paul C. Stomper et al., "Analysis of Parenchymal Density on Mammograms in 1353 Women 25–79 Years Old," *American Journal of Roentgenology* 167, no. 5 (November 1996): 1261–65, https://pubmed.ncbi.nlm.nih.gov/8911192/.

7. "FDA Drug Safety Communication: FDA Warns That

Gadolinium-Based Contrast Agents (GBCAs) Are Retained in the Body; Requires New Class Warnings," US Food & Drug Administration, May 16, 2018, www.fda.gov/drugs /drug-safety-and-availability/fda-drug-safety-communication -fda-warns-gadolinium-based-contrast-agents-gbcas-are -retained-body.

8. Anna N. A. Tosteson et al., "Consequences of False-Positive Screening Mammograms," *JAMA Internal Medicine* 174, no. 6 (June 2014): 954–61, https://www.ncbi.nlm.nih.gov /pmc/articles/PMC4071565/.

9. Nila Alsheik et al., "Outcomes by Race in Breast Cancer Screening with Digital Breast Tomosynthesis versus Digital Mammography," *Journal of the American College of Radiology* 18, no. 7 (July 2021): 906–18, https://pubmed .ncbi.nlm.nih.gov/33607065/.

10. Valentina Silvestri et al., "Characterization of the Cancer Spectrum in Men with Germline BRCA1 and BRCA2 Pathogenic Variants: Results from the Consortium of Investigators of Modifiers of BRCA1/2 (CIMBA)," *JAMA Oncology* 6, no. 8 (August 2020): 1218–30, https://pubmed .ncbi.nlm.nih.gov/32614418/.

11. Donald A. Berry et al., "Effect of Screening and Adjuvant Therapy on Mortality from Breast Cancer," *New England Journal of Medicine* 353, no. 17 (October 2005): 1784–92, https://pubmed.ncbi.nlm.nih.gov/16251534/.

CHAPTER 3: PATHOLOGY, STATE-OF-THE-ART
TREATMENT, AND RECOVERY

1. Osama Alshari et al., "The Effect of Nail Lacquer on Taxane-Induced Nail Changes in Women with Breast Cancer," *Breast Cancer: Basic and Clinical Research (Auckland)* 14 (2020), www.ncbi.nlm.nih.gov/pmc/articles/PMC7297473/.

2. Robert Thomas et al., "A Double-Blind, Randomised Trial
    of a Polyphenolic-Rich Nail Bed Balm for Chemotherapy-
    Induced Onycholysis: The UK Polybalm Study," *Breast
    Cancer Research and Treatment* 171, no. 1 (August 2018):
    103–10, https://pubmed.ncbi.nlm.nih.gov/29736742/.
3. Akiko Hanai et al., "Effects of Cryotherapy on Objective
    and Subjective Symptoms of Paclitaxel-Induced Neuropathy:
    Prospective Self-Controlled Trial," *Journal of the National
    Cancer Institute* 110, no. 2 (February 2018): 141–48,
    https://academic.oup.com/jnci/article/110/2/141/4443215.
4. Weidong Lu et al., "The Value of Acupuncture in Cancer
    Care," *Hematology/Oncology Clinics of North America*
    22, no. 4 (August 2008): 631–48, www.ncbi.nlm.nih.gov
    /pmc/articles/PMC2642987/.
5. Susan Thrane and Susan M. Cohen, "Effect of Reiki
    Therapy on Pain and Anxiety in Adults: An In-Depth
    Literature Review of Randomized Trials with Effect
    Size Calculations," *Pain Management Nursing* 15, no. 4
    (December 2014): 897–908, www.ncbi.nlm.nih.gov/pmc
    /articles/PMC4147026/.

CHAPTER 4: YOU HAVE A GENETIC MUTATION

1. Joi L. Morris and Ora K. Gordon, MD, *Positive Results:
    Making the Best Decisions When You're at High Risk for
    Breast or Ovarian Cancer* (Amherst, NY: Prometheus
    Books, 2010), 45.
2. Mayo Clinic Staff, "BRCA Gene Test for Breast and
    Ovarian Cancer Risk," Mayo Clinic, August 12, 2021,
    www.mayoclinic.org/tests-procedures/brca-gene-test/about
    /pac-20384815.
3. Caroline Helwick, "Dr. Mary-Claire King Proposes
    Population Screening in All Young Women for *BRCA*

Mutations," ASCO Post, February 10, 2015, https://
ascopost.com/issues/february-10-2015/dr-mary-claire-king
-proposes-population-screening-in-all-young-women-for
-brca-mutations/.

4. Luis E. Alvarez, Sebastian D. Eastham, and Steven
   R. H. Barrett, "Radiation Dose to the Global Flying
   Population," *Journal of Radiological Protection* 36, no. 1
   (January 2016): 93–103, https://iopscience.iop.org
   /article/10.1088/0952-4746/36/1/93.

5. "Mammogram Basics," American Cancer Society,
   January 14, 2022, www.cancer.org/cancer/breast-cancer
   /screening-tests-and-early-detection/mammograms
   /mammogram-basics.html.

6. "Radiation Sources and Doses," United States
   Environmental Protection Agency, November 5, 2021,
   www.epa.gov/radiation/radiation-sources-and-doses.

7. "Do You Speak BRCA?" 23andMe.com, www.23andme
   .com/brca/.

8. Holly Yan, "What's the Gene That Led to Angelina Jolie's
   Double Mastectomy?" CNN, May 16, 2013, edition.cnn
   .com/2013/05/14/health/jolie-what-is-brca.

9. Morris and Gordon, *Positive Results*, 45.

10. Elisabeth Jarhelle et al., "Identifying Sequence Variants
    Contributing to Hereditary Breast and Ovarian Cancer in
    BRCA1 and *BRCA2* Negative Breast and Ovarian Cancer
    Patients," *Scientific Reports* 9 (2019): 19986, www.nature
    .com/articles/s41598-019-55515-x.

11. "BRCA Gene Mutations: Cancer Risk and Genetic Testing,"
    National Cancer Institute, November 19, 2020, www
    .cancer.gov/about-cancer/causes-prevention/genetics/brca
    -fact-sheet#what-other-cancers-are-linked-to-harmful
    -variants-in-brca1-and-brca2.

12. Jarhelle et al., "Identifying Sequence Variants."

13. "Genetic Testing," MedlinePlus, https://medlineplus.gov
    /genetictesting.html.

14. Jenni Sheng, "Hormonal Therapy," BreastCancer.org, www
    .breastcancer.org/treatment/hormonal/aromatase_inhibitors.

CHAPTER 5: YOU HAVE AN INCREASED RISK FOR BREAST CANCER

1. "BRCA Exchange Aggregates Data on Thousands of
   BRCA Variants to Inform Understanding of Cancer Risk,"
   news release, National Institutes of Health, January 9,
   2019, www.nih.gov/news-events/news-releases/brca
   -exchange-aggregates-data-thousands-brca-variants-inform
   -understanding-cancer-risk.

2. Michael G. Keeney et al., "Non-*BRCA* Familial Breast
   Cancer: Review of Reported Pathology and Molecular
   Findings," *Pathology* 49, no. 4 (June 2017): 363–70, www
   .sciencedirect.com/science/article/pii/S0031302517300806.

3. "BRCA1 and BRCA2 Gene Mutation Testing &
   Associated Cancers," Memorial Sloan Kettering Cancer
   Center, www.mskcc.org/cancer-care/risk-assessment
   -screening/hereditary-genetics/genetic-counseling/brca1
   -brca2-genes-risk-breast-ovarian.

4. American Cancer Society, *Breast Cancer Facts & Figures
   2019–2020* (Atlanta: American Cancer Society, Inc., 2019),
   www.cancer.org/content/dam/cancer-org/research/cancer
   -facts-and-statistics/breast-cancer-facts-and-figures/breast
   -cancer-facts-and-figures-2019-2020.pdf.

5. Natalie J. Engmann et al., "Population-Attributable Risk
   Proportion of Clinical Risk Factors for Breast Cancer,"
   JAMA Oncology 3, no. 9 (February 2017):1228–36, https://
   jamanetwork.com/journals/jamaoncology/fullarticle/2599991.

6. American College of Radiology, *Breast Imaging Reporting & Data System (BI-RADS) Atlas*, 5th ed. (American College of Radiology, 2013), www.acr.org /Clinical-Resources/Reporting-and-Data-Systems/Bi-Rads.

7. R. D. Rosenberg et al., "Effects of Age, Breast Density, Ethnicity, and Estrogen Replacement Therapy on Screening Mammographic Sensitivity and Cancer Stage at Diagnosis: Review of 183,134 Screening Mammograms in Albuquerque, New Mexico," *Radiology* 209, no. 2 (November 1998): 511–18, https://pubmed.ncbi.nlm.nih.gov/9807581/.

8. Ibid., 518.

9. Pisano et al., "Diagnostic Performance of Digital versus Film Mammography for Breast-Cancer Screening," 1773.

10. Ibid.

11. Norman F. Boyd et al., "Mammographic Density and the Risk and Detection of Breast Cancer," *New England Journal of Medicine* 356, no. 3 (January 2007): 227–36, https://pubmed.ncbi.nlm.nih.gov/17229950/.

12. Stefanie G. A. Veenhuizen et al., "Supplemental Breast MRI for Women with Extremely Dense Breasts: Results of the Second Screening Round of the DENSE Trial," *Radiology* 299, no. 2 (May 2021): 278–86, https://pubs.rsna.org/doi /full/10.1148/radiol.2021203633.

13. "Benign Breast Conditions: Atypical Ductal Hyperplasia," BreastCancer.org, July 27, 2022, www.breastcancer.org /symptoms/benign/atypical-ductal-hyperplasia.

14. Rachel F. Brem et al., "Lobular Neoplasia at Percutaneous Breast Biopsy: Variables Associated with Carcinoma at Surgical Excision," *American Journal of Roentgenology* 190, no. 3 (March 2008): 637–41, https://www.ajronline .org/doi/10.2214/AJR.07.2768.

15. Tari A. King et al., "Lobular Carcinoma in Situ: A 29-Year

Longitudinal Experience Evaluating Clinicopathologic Features and Breast Cancer Risk," *Journal of Clinical Oncology* 33, no. 33 (November 2015): 3945–52, https://www.ncbi.nlm.nih.gov/pmc/articles/PMC4934644/.

16. Lynn C. Hartmann et al., "Atypical Hyperplasia of the Breast—Risk Assessment and Management Options," *New England Journal of Medicine* 372, no. 1 (January 2015): 78–89, https://www.nejm.org/doi/full/10.1056/nejmsr1407164.

17. K. C. Horst et al., "Histologic Subtypes of Breast Cancer Following Radiotherapy for Hodgkin Lymphoma," *Annals of Oncology* 25, no. 4 (April 2014): 848–51, pubmed.ncbi.nlm.nih.gov/24608191/.

18. "Risk Calculator," National Cancer Institute, bcrisktool.cancer.gov/calculator.html.

19. Lucile L. Adams-Campbell et al., "Breast Cancer Risk Assessments Comparing Gail and CARE Models in African-American Women," *Breast Journal* 15, no. 1 (September–October 2009): S72–S75, www.ncbi.nlm.nih.gov/pmc/articles/PMC3760176/.

20. Fernanda Sales Luiz Vianna et al., "Performance of the Gail and Tyrer-Cuzick Breast Cancer Risk Assessment Models in Women Screened in a Primary Care Setting with the FHS-7 Questionnaire," *Genetics and Molecular Biology* 42, supplement 1 (2019): 232–37, www.ncbi.nlm.nih.gov/pmc/articles/PMC6687344/.

21. Catherine Caruso, "Why a Growing Number of Women with Breast Cancer Are Choosing Double Mastectomy," STAT, August 29, 2017, www.statnews.com/2017/08/29/double-mastectomy-breast-cancer/.

22. "Preventive (Prophylactic) Mastectomy: Surgery to Reduce Breast Cancer Risk," Mayo Clinic, January 8, 2021, www

.mayoclinic.org/tests-procedures/mastectomy/in-depth
/prophylactic-mastectomy/art-20047221.

23. Catherine E. Pesce et al., "Changing Surgical Trends in
Young Patients with Early Stage Breast Cancer, 2003 to
2010: A Report from the National Cancer Data Base,"
Journal of the American College of Surgeons 219, no. 1
(July 2014): 19–28, pubmed.ncbi.nlm.nih.gov/24862886/.

24. Reshma Jagsi et al., "Contralateral Prophylactic
Mastectomy Decisions in a Population-Based Sample of
Patients with Early-Stage Breast Cancer," *JAMA Surgery*
152, no. 3 (2017): 274–82, jamanetwork.com/journals
/jamasurgery/article-abstract/2593807.

25. Amanda K. Arrington et al., "Patient and Surgeon
Characteristics Associated with Increased Use of Contralateral
Prophylactic Mastectomy in Patients with Breast Cancer,"
Annals of Surgical Oncology 16, no. 10 (October 2009):
2697–704, pubmed.ncbi.nlm.nih.gov/19653045/.

26. Sarah T. Hawley et al., "The Association between Patient
Attitudes and Values and the Strength of Consideration for
Contralateral Prophylactic Mastectomy in a Population-
Based Sample of Breast Cancer Patients," *Cancer* 123
(2017): 4547–55, acsjournals.onlinelibrary.wiley.com/doi
/full/10.1002/cncr.30924.

27. Caruso, "Why a Growing Number of Women with Breast
Cancer Are Choosing Double Mastectomy."

28. Ibid.

CHAPTER 6: YOU HAVE BREAST CANCER AT A YOUNG AGE

1. Carey K. Anders et al., "Young Age at Diagnosis
Correlates with Worse Prognosis and Defines a Subset
of Breast Cancers with Shared Patterns of Gene
Expression," *Journal of Clinical Oncology* 26, no. 20

(July 2008): 3324–30, ascopubs.org/doi/10.1200 /JCO.2007.14.2471.

2. Ann H. Partridge, Aron Goldhirsch, Shari Gelber, and Richard D. Gelber, "Breast Cancer in Younger Women," in Jay R. Harris, Marc E. Lippman, Monica Morrow, and C. Kent Osborne, eds., *Diseases of the Breast*, 5th ed. (Philadelphia: Wolters Kluwer, 2014), 1101–11.

3. Colleen Moriarty, "Too Young to Screen: Breast Cancer in Younger Women," Yale Medicine, September 28, 2020, www.yalemedicine.org/news/breast-cancer-younger -women.

4. "Breast Cancer Statistics in Young Adults," Young Survival Coalition, www.youngsurvival.org/learn/about-breast -cancer/statistics.

5. Rebecca H. Johnson, Franklin L. Chien, and Archie Bleyer, "Incidence of Breast Cancer with Distant Involvement among Women in the United States, 1976 to 2009," *JAMA* 309, no. 8 (2013): 800–805, jamanetwork.com/journals /jama/fullarticle/1656255.

6. K. J. Ruddy et al., "Presentation of Breast Cancer in Young Women," *Journal of Clinical Oncology* 27, no. 15, supplement (2009): 6608, ascopubs.org/doi/abs/10.1200 /jco.2009.27.15_suppl.6608.

7. "Five Things Women under 40 Should Know about Breast Cancer," Beth Israel Deaconsess Medical Center, September 30, 2019, www.bidmc.org/about-bidmc/wellness -insights/breast-health/2019/09/five-things-women-under -40-should-know-about-breast-cancer.

8. American Cancer Society, *Breast Cancer Facts & Figures 2015–2016* (Atlanta: American Cancer Society, Inc., 2015).

9. Alexandra W. van den Belt-Dusebout et al., "Ovarian Stimulation for In Vitro Fertilization and Long-Term Risk of

Breast Cancer," *JAMA* 316, no. 3 (2016): 300–312, https://jamanetwork.com/journals/jama/fullarticle/2533505.

10. Youlia M. Kirova et al., "Risk of Breast Cancer Recurrence and Contralateral Breast Cancer in Relation to *BRCA1* and *BRCA2* Mutation Status following Breast-Conserving Surgery and Radiotherapy," *European Journal of Cancer* 41, no. 15 (October 2005): 2304–11, https://doi.org/10.1016/j.ejca.2005.02.037.

11. Kelly Metcalfe et al., "Risk of Ipsilateral Breast Cancer in BRCA1 and BRCA2 Mutation Carriers," *Breast Cancer Research and Treatment* 127 (2011): 287–96, https://doi.org/10.1007/s10549-010-1336-7.

12. Harry Bartelink et al., "Recurrence Rates after Treatment of Breast Cancer with Standard Radiotherapy with or without Additional Radiation," *New England Journal of Medicine* 345, no. 19 (November 2001): 1378–87, https://pubmed.ncbi.nlm.nih.gov/11794170/.

13. Jagsi et al., "Contralateral Prophylactic Mastectomy Decisions," 282.

14. Moriarty, "Too Young to Screen."

15. Ann H. Partridge et al., "Age of Menopause among Women Who Remain Premenopausal following Treatment for Early Breast Cancer: Long-Term Results from International Breast Cancer Study Group Trials V and VI," *European Journal of Cancer* 43, no. 11 (July 2007): 1646–53, https://www.sciencedirect.com/science/article/abs/pii/S0959804907002912.

16. "NCCN Guidelines: Breast Cancer," National Comprehensive Cancer Network, https://www.nccn.org/guidelines/guidelines-detail?category=1&id=1419.

17. Partridge et al., "Age of Menopause," 1653.

18. Anna Marklund et al., "Reproductive Outcomes after

Breast Cancer in Women with vs without Fertility
Preservation," *JAMA Oncology* 7, no. 1 (January 2021):
86–91, https://pubmed.ncbi.nlm.nih.gov/33211089/.

19. Mayo Clinic Staff, "Egg Freezing," Mayo Clinic, April 23,
2021, www.mayoclinic.org/tests-procedures/egg-freezing
/about/pac-20384556.

20. "Treating Breast Cancer during Pregnancy," American
Cancer Society, October 27, 2021, www.cancer.org/cancer
/breast-cancer/treatment/treating-breast-cancer-during
-pregnancy.html.

21. Eryn B. Callihan et al., "Postpartum Diagnosis
Demonstrates a High Risk for Metastasis and Merits an
Expanded Definition of Pregnancy-Associated Breast
Cancer," *Breast Cancer Research and Treatment* 138,
no. 2 (2013): 549–59, www.ncbi.nlm.nih.gov/pmc/articles
/PMC3608871/.

22. "Treating Breast Cancer during Pregnancy."

23. Ibid.

24. Ibid.

25. Jamie DePolo, "Surgery Choice for Early-Stage Breast
Cancer Seems to Affect Younger Women's Quality of Life,"
BreastCancer.org, September 26, 2022, www.breastcancer
.org/research-news/early-stage-sx-choice-affects-young
-womens-qol.

26. Kate O'Rourke, "Young Women with Breast Cancer
Pursue Aggressive Surgery," Clinical Oncology News,
April 19, 2019, www.clinicaloncology.com/Breast-Cancer
/Article/04-19/Young-Women-With-Breast-Cancer-Pursue
-Aggressive-Surgery/54597.

27. K. Rojas et al., "The Impact of Mastectomy Type on the
Female Sexual Function Index (FSFI), Satisfaction with
Appearance, and the Reconstructed Breast's Role in

Intimacy," *Breast Cancer Research and Treatment* 163, no. 2 (June 2017): 273–79, pubmed.ncbi.nlm.nih .gov/28260139/; and Jesse T. Casaubon et al., "Breast-Specific Sensuality and Appearance Satisfaction: Comparison of Breast-Conserving Surgery and Nipple-Sparing Mastectomy," *Journal of the American College of Surgeons* 230, no. 6 (June 2020): 990–98, pubmed.ncbi .nlm.nih.gov/32272205/.

28. DePolo, "Surgery Choice for Early-Stage Breast Cancer."
29. Ibid.
30. Nora E. Carbine et al., "Risk-Reducing Mastectomy for the Prevention of Primary Breast Cancer," *Cochrane Database of Systematic Reviews*, 2019, https://www.cochranelibrary .com/cdsr/doi/10.1002/14651858.CD002748.pub4/full.
31. Brian Wojciechowski, "More Evidence That Chemotherapy before Surgery Can Make Triple-Negative Breast Cancer Eligible for Lumpectomy," BreastCancer.org, January 15, 2020, www.breastcancer.org/research-news/chemo-before -sx-makes-tnbc-eligible-for-lx.
32. "Ask the Cancer Genetics Team: Medical and Psychological Considerations of a Preventive Mastectomy," Dana-Farber Cancer Institute, www .dana-farber.org/health-library/articles/ask-the -cancer-genetics-team—medical-and-psychological -considerations-of-a-preventive-mastectomy/.
33. "Does Having Preventive Mastectomy Improve Quality of Life?" BreastCancer.org, July 31, 2022, www.breastcancer .org/research-news/does-preventive-mx-improve-qol.

CHAPTER 7: YOU HAVE POSTMENOPAUSAL BREAST CANCER

1. Rosemary Yancik et al., "Effect of Age and Comorbidity in Post-Menopausal Breast Cancer Patients Aged 55 Years and

Older," *JAMA* 285, no. 7 (2001): 885–92, jamanetwork
.com/journals/jama/fullarticle/193570.

2. Nam P. Nguyen et al., "Older Breast Cancer
   Undertreatment: Unconscious Bias to Undertreat—Potential
   Role for the International Geriatric Radiotherapy Group?"
   Translational Cancer Research 9, supplement 1 (January
   2020), www.ncbi.nlm.nih.gov/pmc/articles/PMC2894028/.

3. Barbara Stepko, "Breast Cancer after Menopause," AARP,
   October 3, 2018, www.aarp.org/health/conditions
   -treatments/info-2018/breast-cancer-after-menopause.html.

4. Laura Nathan-Garner, "How Does Menopause Affect
   Cancer Risk?" MD Anderson Cancer Center, November
   2015, www.mdanderson.org/publications/focused-on
   -health/FOH-menopause-cancer.h20-1589835.html.

5. Ibid.

6. Ibid.

7. Stepko, "Breast Cancer after Menopause."

8. Victoria Tang et al., "Functional Status and Survival after
   Breast Cancer Surgery in Nursing Home Residents," *JAMA
   Surgery* 153, no. 12 (2018): 1090–96, https://jamanetwork
   .com/journals/jamasurgery/fullarticle/2697211.

9. Ibid., 1096.

10. Yancik et al., "Effect of Age," 892.

11. Ibid.

12. "Breast Cancer Deaths Down 40% Since 1990, Thanks
    to Mammography," Radiology Business, March 31, 2017,
    www.radiologybusiness.com/topics/care-optimization
    /breast-cancer-deaths-down-40-1990-thanks-mammography.

CHAPTER 8: YOUR MASTECTOMY OPTIONS

1. Elisa Port, MD, *The New Generation Breast Cancer
   Book: How to Navigate Your Diagnosis and Treatment*

Options—and Remain Optimistic—in an Age of Information Overload (New York: Ballantine, 2015), 81.

2. Caruso, "Why a Growing Number of Women with Breast Cancer Are Choosing Double Mastectomy."

3. Ibid.

4. Susan M. Domchek et al., "Association of Risk-Reducing Surgery in BRCA1 or BRCA2 Mutation Carriers with Cancer Risk and Mortality," *JAMA* 304, no. 9 (September 2010): 967–75, pubmed.ncbi.nlm.nih.gov/20810374/.

5. Caruso, "Why a Growing Number of Women with Breast Cancer Are Choosing Double Mastectomy."

6. Monica J. Smith, "No Benefit of Contralateral Prophylactic Mastectomy in Most Cancer Patients," General Surgery News, October 8, 2018, www.generalsurgerynews.com /In-the-News/Article/10-18/No-Benefit-of-Contralateral -Prophylactic-Mastectomy-in-Most-Cancer-Patients/53015?s ub=C1482AB761B48AE85DE98ACDD4FBEDFB118F0E7E B1EEE62DA06F6B3F3476D9&enl=true.

7. Kristine Conner, "Going Flat after Mastectomy," BreastCancer.org, October 3, 2022, www .breastcancer.org/treatment/surgery/reconstruction/no -reconstruction.

8. Jennifer L. Baker et al., "'Going Flat' after Mastectomy: Patient-Reported Outcomes by Online Survey," *Annals of Surgical Oncology* 28 (2021): 2493–505, https://link .springer.com/article/10.1245/s10434-020-09448-9.

9. Howard N. Langstein et al., "Breast Cancer Recurrence after Immediate Reconstruction: Patterns and Significance," *Plastic and Reconstructive Surgery* 111, no. 2 (February 2003): 712–20, journals.lww.com/plasreconsurg/Abstract /2003/02000/Breast_Cancer_Recurrence_after_Immediate .32.aspx.

10. "ASBrS 2018: Modern Therapies Minimize Recurrence after Breast-Conserving Surgery," ASCO Post, May 8, 2018, ascopost.com/News/58821.

11. Bernadette A. M. Heemskerk-Gerritsen et al., "Survival after Bilateral Risk-Reducing Mastectomy in Healthy BRCA1 and BRCA2 Mutation Carriers," *Breast Cancer Research and Treatment* 177, no. 3 (2019): 723–33, www.ncbi.nlm.nih.gov/pmc/articles/PMC6745043/.

12. Kelly Metcalfe et al., "Contralateral Mastectomy and Survival after Breast Cancer in Carriers of BRCA1 and BRCA2 Mutations: Retrospective Analysis," *BMJ* 348 (2014): g226, www.ncbi.nlm.nih.gov/pmc/articles/PMC3921438/.

13. Toni Musiello, Emelie Bornhammar, and Christobel Saunders, "Breast Surgeons' Perceptions and Attitudes towards Contralateral Prophylactic Mastectomy," *ANZ Journal of Surgery* 83, nos. 7–8 (July 2013): 527–32, pubmed.ncbi.nlm.nih.gov/23043449/.

14. Jessica Gahm, Marie Wickman, and Yvonne Brandberg, "Bilateral Prophylactic Mastectomy in Women with Inherited Risk of Breast Cancer—Prevalence of Pain and Discomfort, Impact on Sexuality, Quality of Life and Feelings of Regret Two Years after Surgery," *Breast* 19, no. 6 (December 2010): 462–69, pubmed.ncbi.nlm.nih.gov/20605453/.

CHAPTER 9: YOUR NEW BREASTS

1. Jennifer Harrington, MD, "Why Today's Breast Augmentation Is Better than Ever," *Connect* (blog), American Society of Plastic Surgeons, July 17, 2018, www.plasticsurgery.org/news/blog/why-todays-breast-augmentation-is-better-than-ever.

2. Sawyer Cimaroli, John A. LoGiudice, and Erin L. Doren, "Exploring the Role of Partner Satisfaction in Predicting Patient Satisfaction Regarding Post-Mastectomy Breast Reconstruction," *Plastic and Reconstructive Surgery Global Open* 8, no. 7 (July 2020): e2943, https://www.ncbi.nlm .nih.gov/pmc/articles/PMC7413778/.

3. Charlotte Bath, "Breast Reconstruction: 'A Process, Not a Procedure' with Potential Short- and Long-Term Complications," ASCO Post, August 25, 2018, ascopost .com/issues/august-25-2018/breast-reconstruction/.

4. Joshua C. Doloff et al., "The Surface Topography of Silicone Breast Implants Mediates the Foreign Body Response in Mice, Rabbits, and Humans," *Nature Biomedical Engineering* 5 (2021): 1115–30, https://doi .org/10.1038/s41551-021-00739-4.

5. "Tug Flap Breast Reconstruction," Barnes Jewish Hospital, www.barnesjewish.org/Medical-Services/Plastic -Reconstructive-Surgery/Breast-Reconstruction/TUG-Flap -Breast-Reconstruction.

6. "Types of Breast Reconstruction," BreastCancer.org, June 29, 2022, www.breastcancer.org/treatment/surgery /reconstruction/types/.

CHAPTER 10: HOW YOUR LOVED ONES CAN HELP

1. "Cara Scharf," GW Cancer Center, cancercenter.gwu.edu /profile/patient/cara-scharf.

2. "Family and Friends: Support for Family, Friends, and Caregivers," Cancer Support Community, www .cancersupportcommunity.org/friends-family.

3. Adam Hinzey et al., "Breast Cancer and Social Environment: Getting By with a Little Help from Our Friends," *Breast Cancer Research* 18, no. 1 (May 2016): 54,

https://pubmed.ncbi.nlm.nih.gov/27225892/; and Fatemeh Moghaddam Tabrizi, Moloud Radfar, and Zeynab Taei, "Effects of Supportive-Expressive Discussion Groups on Loneliness, Hope, and Quality of Life in Breast Cancer Survivors: A Randomized Control Trial," *Psycho-Oncology* 25, no. 9 (September 2016): 1057–63, https://pubmed.ncbi.nlm.nih.gov/27302306/.

CHAPTER 11: THE FUTURE

1. K. C. Chu, C. R. Smart, and R. E. Tarone, "Analysis of Breast Cancer Mortality and Stage Distribution by Age for the Health Insurance Plan Clinical Trial," *Journal of the National Cancer Institute* 80, no. 14 (September 1988): 1125–32, https://pubmed.ncbi.nlm.nih.gov/3411625/.

2. Allie Nawrat, "Breast Cancer Timeline: Charting Three Decades of Success," Pharmaceutical Technology, December 19, 2019, www.pharmaceutical-technology.com /features/bresat-cancer-charting-success/.

3. Rena Goldman, "History of Breast Cancer," Healthline, December 30, 2020, www.healthline.com/health/history-of -breast-cancer.

4. Nawrat, "Breast Cancer Timeline."

5. Goldman, "History of Breast Cancer."

6. "The Ground We've Gained," Breast Cancer Research Foundation, www.bcrf.org/breast-cancer-research -breakthroughs/.

7. Nawrat, "Breast Cancer Timeline."

8. "The Ground We've Gained."

9. Nawrat, "Breast Cancer Timeline."

10. "The Ground We've Gained."

11. Ibid.

12. Ibid.

13. Goldman, "History of Breast Cancer."

14. "What Is Personalized Cancer Medicine?" Cancer.net, www.cancer.net/navigating-cancer-care/how-cancer-treated /personalized-and-targeted-therapies/what-personalized -cancer-medicine.

15. Ibid.

16. Marthe Larsen et al., "Artificial Intelligence Evaluation of 122,969 Mammography Examinations from a Population- Based Screening Program," *Radiology* 303, no. 3 (March 2022): 502–11, https://pubs.rsna.org/doi/epdf/10.1148 /radiol.212381.

17. José Luis Raya-Povedano et al., "AI-Based Strategies to Reduce Workload in Breast Cancer Screening with Mammography and Tomosynthesis: A Retrospective Evaluation," *Radiology* 300, no. 1 (July 2021): 57–65, https://pubs.rsna.org/doi/full/10.1148/radiol.2021203555.

18. Dominique Sighoko et al., "Changes in the Racial Disparity in Breast Cancer Mortality in the Ten US Cities with the Largest African American Populations from 1999 to 2013: The Reduction in Breast Cancer Mortality Disparity in Chicago," *Cancer Causes & Control* 28, no. 6 (June 2017): 563–68, https://www.ncbi.nlm.nih.gov/pmc/articles /PMC5400784/.

19. Maneet Kaur et al., "Trends in Breast Cancer Incidence Rates by Race/Ethnicity: Patterns by Stage, Socioeconomic Position, and Geography in the United States, 1999–2017," *Cancer* 128, no. 5 (March 2022): 1015–23, https:// acsjournals.onlinelibrary.wiley.com/doi/abs/10.1002 /cncr.34008.

20. Raya-Povedano et al., "AI-Based Strategies to Reduce Workload," 65.

21. Tomonori Kanda et al., "Distribution and Chemical Forms

of Gadolinium in the Brain: A Review," *British Journal of Radiology* 90, no. 1079 (November 2017): 20170115, https://www.ncbi.nlm.nih.gov/pmc/articles/PMC5963376/.

22. "Delphinus Receives FDA Approval for Its SoftVue 3D Whole Breast Ultrasound Tomography System," press release, Delphinus Medical Technologies, October 12, 2021, delphinusmt.com/news/delphinus-receives-fda-approval-for -its-softvue-3d-whole-breast-ultrasound-tomography-system/.

23. Neb Duric et al., "Using Whole Breast Ultrasound Tomography to Improve Breast Cancer Risk Assessment: A Novel Risk Factor Based on the Quantitative Tissue Property of Sound Speed," *Journal of Clinical Medicine* 9, no. 2 (January 2020): 367, https://pubmed.ncbi.nlm.nih .gov/32013177/.

24. Edoardo Botteri et al., "Modeling the Relationship between Circulating Tumour Cells Number and Prognosis of Metastatic Breast Cancer," *Breast Cancer Research and Treatment* 122, no. 1 (July 2010): 211–17, https://pubmed .ncbi.nlm.nih.gov/19967556/.

25. Olena Weaver and Jessica W. T. Leung, "Biomarkers and Imaging of Breast Cancer," *American Journal of Roentgenology* 210, no. 2 (February 2018): 271–78, https:// pubmed.ncbi.nlm.nih.gov/29166151/.

26. George H. Sakorafas et al., "Lymphedema following Axillary Lymph Node Dissection for Breast Cancer," *Surgical Oncology* 15, no. 3 (November 2006): 153–65, https://pubmed.ncbi.nlm.nih.gov/17187979/.

27. Anna Rose Johnson et al., "Evaluating the Impact of Immediate Lymphatic Reconstruction for the Surgical Prevention of Lymphedema," *Plastic and Reconstructive Surgery* 147, no. 3 (March 2021): 373e–81e, https://pubmed .ncbi.nlm.nih.gov/33620920/.

28. Michelle Coriddi et al., "Immediate Lymphatic Reconstruction: Technical Points and Literature Review," *Plastic and Reconstructive Surgery Global Open* 9, no. 2 (February 2021): e3431, https://pubmed.ncbi.nlm.nih .gov/33680675/.

29. Reshma Jagsi et al., "Radiation Field Design in the ACOSOG Z0011 (Alliance) Trial," *Journal of Clinical Oncology* 32, no. 32 (November 2014): 3600–3606, https:// pubmed.ncbi.nlm.nih.gov/25135994/; and S. R. Tee et al., "Meta-Analysis of Sentinel Lymph Node Biopsy after Neoadjuvant Chemotherapy in Patients with Initial Biopsy-Proven Node-Positive Breast Cancer," *British Journal of Surgery* 105, no. 12 (November 2018): 1541–52, https:// pubmed.ncbi.nlm.nih.gov/30311642/.

30. Brianna Majsiak, "What Is a Sensation Preserving Mastectomy?" Everyday Health, October 28, 2021, www .everydayhealth.com/breast-cancer/what-is-a-sensation -preserving-mastectomy/.

31. Kristy L. Hamilton, Katarzyna E. Kania, and Aldona J. Spiegel, "Post-Mastectomy Sensory Recovery and Restoration," *Gland Surgery* 10, no. 1 (January 2021): 494–97, www.ncbi.nlm.nih.gov/pmc/articles/PMC7882309/; Anne Warren Peled and Ziv M. Peled, "Nerve Preservation and Allografting for Sensory Innervation following Immediate Implant Breast Reconstruction," *Plastic Reconstructive Surgery Global Open* 7, no. 7 (July 2019): e2332, www.ncbi.nlm.nih.gov/pmc/articles/PMC6952160/; and Jacob R. Burns, Tatyana S. Polyak, and Clifford T. Pereira, "Neurotization of the Nipple-Areola Complex during Implant-Based Reconstruction: Evaluation of Early Sensation Recovery," *Plastic and Reconstructive Surgery* 148, no. 1 (July 2021): 143e–44e.

32. Catherine F. Cowell et al., "Progression from Ductal Carcinoma *In Situ* to Invasive Breast Cancer: Revisited," *Molecular Oncology* 7, no. 5 (October 2013): 859–69, www.ncbi.nlm.nih.gov/pmc/articles/PMC5528459/.

33. E. Shelley Hwang et al., "The COMET (Comparison of Operative versus Monitoring and Endocrine Therapy) Trial: A Phase III Randomised Controlled Clinical Trial for Low-Risk Ductal Carcinoma In Situ (DCIS)," *BMJ Open* 9, no. 3 (March 2019): e026797, https://www.ncbi.nlm.nih.gov/pmc/articles/PMC6429899/.

34. Maartje van Seijen et al., "Ductal Carcinoma In Situ: To Treat or Not to Treat, That Is the Question," *British Journal of Cancer* 121 (July 2019): 285–92, www.nature.com/articles/s41416-019-0478-6.

Index

About the Authors

DR. RACHEL BREM is an internationally known breast cancer expert. She is a professor and the vice chairwoman of the department of radiology and the director of breast imaging and intervention at the George Washington University School of Medicine & Health Sciences. Dr. Brem is on the boards of directors of numerous industry-leading companies and is the chief medical advisor and cofounder of the Brem Foundation. Dr. Brem is a fellow of the American College of Radiology and the Society of Breast Imaging and is the recipient of many awards, including being named a *Newsweek* Best Cancer Doctor, a Castle Connolly Top Doctor, and a Castle Connolly Top Cancer Doctor in the United States.

DR. CHRISTY TEAL is an associate professor of surgery, the director of the Breast Care Center, and chief of breast surgery at the George Washington University School of Medicine & Health Sciences. Dr. Teal and her colleagues have developed a cutting-edge, holistic, patient-focused Breast Care Center that integrates complementary medicine with the latest technology and surgical innovations. She is a fellow of the American College of Surgeons and a member of the American Society of Breast Surgeons, a *Washingtonian* Top Doctor, a Castle Connolly Top Doctor, and a Castle Connolly Exceptional Women in Medicine award recipient.